BLACK WELLNESS BARRIERS

BLACK WELLNESS BARRIERS

*Understanding the Root Cause of Disease
Vulnerabilities as a Pathway Towards Restoring Health*

Dr. Tawainna Houston

Black Wellness Barriers: Understanding The Root Cause Of Disease Vulnerabilities As A Pathway Towards Restoring Health

Copyright © 2025 by Tawainna D. Houston

All rights reserved, no part of this publication may be reproduced, distributed, or transmitted in any form, by any means electronic or mechanical, including photocopying, recording, or by any information storage retrieval system, without permission in writing from the author, except for the inclusion of brief quotations and certain other noncommercial uses permitted by copyright law. For permission requests contact: support@blackcellconsulting.com

Black CELL Consulting, LLC
2510 East Sunset Rd. Ste 5-924
Las Vegas, NV 89120

First Edition: August 2025

Special discounts are available for bulk purchases of this book for business, educational, or promotional use. For more information, please contact: support@blackcellconsulting.com

DISCLAIMER:

The information written in this book is based on the education, research, and experience of the author and is therefore not intended to replace visits to a licensed healthcare professional. The information in this book is not intended to diagnose, treat, or cure any medical condition. This information is intended as a resource for health information, to be used in conjunction with your visits to qualified healthcare professionals.

ISBN : 979-8-9995165-0-3

Library of Congress Control Number: 2025914801

Printed in the United States of America

This book is dedicated to all the known and unknown, named and unnamed ancestors whose blood, sweat, and tears paved the way. Because of you, we exist to remember your story, tell your story, honor your legacy, and continue to build upon it.

CONTENTS

Introduction Context Is the Key   9

Author's Note: 15

PART I: HISTORICAL FOUNDATIONS OF DEHUMANIZATION   17

    Chapter 1: The Myth of Inferiority: The Origin Story   20

    Chapter 2: Embodied Exploitation: The Physical Toll of Slavery on Black Health   38

    Chapter 3: The Psychological Assault: Trauma, Control, and Identity Erasure   56

PART II STRUCTURAL BARRIERS TO WELLNESS   82

    Barrier One: Housing and the Geography of Injustice   83

    Barrier Two: Education as a Gatekeeper to Opportunity   88

    Barrier Three: Food Apartheid and Nutritional Access   95

    Barrier Four: Healthcare Denial, Delay, and Dismissal   99

    Barrier Five: Labor Inequity and Economic Fragility   105

    Barrier Six: Socioeconomic Disadvantage   112

    Barrier Seven: Environmental Racism and Toxic Exposures   117

Barrier Eight: Safety and Surveillance 123

Barrier Nine: Transportation as an Obstacle to Wellness 128

Barrier Ten: Identity and Stigma in Public Spaces 131

PART III: THE BIOLOGY OF OPPRESSION **139**

Chapter 4: Under Pressure: Chronic Stress and
the Lived Black Experience 142

Chapter 5: Epigenetics and Ancestral Imprints:
The Biology of Inherited Trauma 162

Part IV: RECLAIMING BLACK WELLNESS **176**

Chapter 6: The Collectivism of Wellness 179

Principle One: Umoja (Unity) 192

Principle Two: Kujichagulia (Self-Determination) 196

Principle Three: Ujima (Collective Work and Responsibility) 200

Principle Four: Ujamaa (Cooperative Economics) 204

Principle Five: Nia (Purpose) 208

Principle Six: Kuumba (Creativity) 212

Principle Seven: Imani (Faith) 217

Chapter 7: The 12 Key Elements of Individualized Wellness:
Tools for Black Health & Longevity 223

Element 1—Breath: Grounding in the Present 225

Element 2—Hydration: Nourishing the Inner Landscape 229

Element 3—Nutrition: Reclaiming Food as Medicine 234

Element 4–Movement: Reconnecting to Strength & Vitality	239
Element 5–Circulation: Stimulating Vital Flow	244
Element 6–Digestion: The Root of Health and Disease	249
Element 7–Detoxification: Cleansing Toxins as a Lifestyle	254
Element 8 – Rest: Sacred Stillness and Renewal	259
Element 9 – Inflammation Regulation: Reducing the Body's Alarm System	263
Element 10 – Immune System Protection: Strengthening the Body's Defense	268
Element 11 – Stress Management: Cultivating Calm in a Chaotic World	273
Element 12 – Connection: Building Belonging and Safe Space	278
Bonus Element – Prevention Is Power: Taking Charge Before Disease Takes Hold	283
Conclusion	**294**
Acknowledgements	**298**
Endnotes	**299**
Index	**323**
About The Author	**331**

INTRODUCTION
CONTEXT IS THE KEY: REFRAMING BLACK HEALTH THROUGH A HISTORICAL LENS

Context is where it all begins, or at least where it should begin. In our daily lives, we instinctively look to context when tragedy strikes—when the unthinkable happens. Our minds become restless without a backstory, a cause, or something to explain the seemingly unfathomable. This insatiable curiosity—the drive to get to the bottom of things—often seems to be missing when it comes to the health of African Americans. Statistics showing Black people die younger, sicker, and more often are presented as fact, unchallenged, and decontextualized. The human instinct to seek meaning via context is lost here. "It is what it is" seems to be the ethos accepted as the status quo regarding Black health.

I can vividly remember sitting in a medical school lecture as my white male professor noted, almost casually, that hypertension is more common in Black patients. It was that simple, a bullet point on a slide. "Be mindful of this when treating Black patients," he said. It wasn't new information—I had heard versions of it for years. Black people have higher rates of diabetes. Black people are more likely to have strokes. Black women are more likely to be overweight. That particular day, in that lecture hall, the familiar refrain hit differently. I was suddenly filled with a quiet rage. Again, we were being defined by what ails us, without explaining WHY. The focus was solely on the data. No history. No mention of lived experience. No acknowledgment of the systems that have shaped our reality.

What enraged me most was the ease with which this narrative was delivered, as though disease in the Black body was natural, inevitable, and self-inflicted. The room of my majority white classmates didn't pause to ask why. No one seemed to consider that this presentation of the "what" without the "why" was not only incomplete but dangerous. Without context, an old and insidious narrative emerges: the lie of Black biological inferiority.

That lie, rooted in slavery, protected by policy, and echoed in medicine, continues to shape how we as Black people are seen and how we see ourselves. Most dangerously, it erodes the collective ability to imagine something different: a future where Black bodies aren't blamed for their own suffering; more importantly, a future where the structural and interpersonal conditions that created our suffering are interrogated, dismantled, and healed.

Black Wellness Barriers: Understanding the Root Cause of Disease Vulnerabilities as a Pathway Towards Restoring Health is not just a book—it's a long-overdue reckoning. It's an effort to tell the full story with broad strokes of how we got here and why we carry such a heavy burden of disease. This is not a book about blame—it's a book about truth. And more importantly, it's a book about power. The power we hold when we stop normalizing our pain, stop minimizing our history, and start naming what has been done to us.

This book is anchored in four fundamental elements that together create a framework for understanding the health vulnerabilities faced by Black Americans: *historical dehumanization, structural barriers, stress response, and transgenerational trauma.* These are not abstract theories—they are the lived realities that have shaped every generation since the first Africans were brought to this land in chains.

We begin with history—American history—not because we are stuck in the past, but because the past is still alive in our bodies. Enslavement wasn't just a moral failing. It was a system that commodified Black bodies, stripped away personhood, and subjected people to brutal physical and psychological abuse for generations. Our ancestors were not allowed to own their bodies, let alone tend to their health. Malnourishment, medical experimentation, forced reproduction, and denial of care were daily realities. These were not isolated acts of cruelty—they were legalized, normalized, and even justified through pseudoscientific lies that Black people felt less pain, needed less rest, and were biologically suited for servitude.

These beliefs didn't end with emancipation. They mutated. In the post-slavery era, Black communities were systematically excluded from healthcare systems by being pushed into segregated hospitals and neglected by public health infrastructure. This exclusion was not incidental but policy-based. It laid the foundation for the disparities we now call "inequities."

The reality is that this is not just about what was done to our ancestors. It is about what continues to happen today. Our bodies are still bearing the weight of centuries of accumulated stress. Structural racism isn't just a political concept—it's a physiological reality. When you live in an environment that constantly devalues your humanity at every turn, your body responds. It stays on alert. It fights to survive. That fight takes a toll on the heart, the immune system, and mental health. This constant wear and tear, or allostatic load, becomes its own health condition over time. Unfortunately, it is a condition directly linked to the diseases that disproportionately claim Black lives.

This stress doesn't end with one generation. It gets passed down. We now have scientific evidence—through the study of epigenetics—that trauma can leave biological footprints across generations. Our genes don't change, but the way they express themselves can be impacted. This is how the trauma of enslavement, Jim Crow, and modern systemic racism continues to echo through our bodies today. Transgenerational trauma is not just a psychological concept; it is a biological inheritance.

And yet, we are so often told to move on. To stop talking about the past. To stop "acting like victims." But let's be clear—naming pain is not weakness; it is strength. It is the first and most necessary step toward healing. We cannot bypass discomfort simply because it's easier to pretend everything is fine. We cannot continue suppressing our hurts with the belief that we are denying white people the satisfaction of triggering our emotions. We cannot keep silencing ourselves because we are tired of having to justify our truth. Healing cannot happen without truth, and truth cannot exist without context.

The truth is that the enslavement of our ancestors was a crime against humanity. Where there are crimes, there are victims and there are perpetrators. Victims experience harm, injury, and loss—often at the hands of those who will never be held accountable. Instead of acknowledging that truth, mainstream society has too often condemned the Black community for even daring to whisper the echoes of that collective pain.

Introduction

As a result, that pain has been buried, distorted, and turned inward. For many, it becomes an internalized shame. For others, it breeds denial—the mistaken belief that history is irrelevant or best left untouched. Avoidance does not serve us. To fully sit with the reality of what happened to our ancestors, what still reverberates in us today, can feel overwhelming, even unbearable. And yet, the only way out is through.

I know these pages won't be easy to read. There will be moments of discomfort. Perhaps even grief. Keep going. Sit with what hurts. On the other side of the truth is possibility. Despite all we've endured, we are still here. We are still building, still resisting, still loving, still culturally healing. That is not a small thing. That is legacy. And it deserves to be protected.

This book will examine the historical, structural, and biological forces that have shaped Black health and provide pathways forward. There are collective and individual strategies that we can adopt and cultural frameworks to be reclaimed. While we didn't create these conditions, we have the power to respond to them with intention and clarity. We have the ability to write a different story.

Society has treated Black health like a trend, only prioritizing it during pandemics or after public outcries. We don't need permission to care about our wellness. We don't need another crisis like COVID-19 colliding with the murder of George Floyd to prove that Black Lives Matter. We matter now. We always have, and so do our futures.

This book is written for us, but it is also written with others in mind. For the policymakers, scholars, and medical practitioners who say they care about equity, here is your context. For well-meaning allies who want to understand why we are angry, why we are tired, and why we are still fighting: read closely. For every Black reader who has ever felt unseen, unheard, or unwell, this book is a mirror and a map.

We cannot heal what we refuse to name. And we cannot thrive without understanding how we've survived. The time for survival-only living is over. Now, we write a new chapter, one rooted in truth, wellness, and liberation.

AUTHOR'S NOTE:

———

Black Wellness Barriers

Throughout Black Wellness Barriers, I use the terms African American, Black, and Black American interchangeably. I recognize, however, that not all Black people in the U.S. are descendants of enslaved Africans in America. Our collective history is vast, layered, and shaped by differing historical realities. As such, some of the historical context in Part I may not directly apply to Black Americans from other parts of the diaspora.

Still, as this book will show, second- and third-generation Black immigrants often encounter similar stress-induced cellular changes that African Americans have endured for generations. While cultural and social experiences across the diaspora differ, America offers one limiting box in which we are all perceived, judged, and often discriminated against. Tragically, this imposed social hierarchy has conditioned many of us to judge one another based on origin rather than honoring our shared struggles and cultural strengths.

I understand—no one wants to be placed at the bottom of the totem pole. But even if that's where we were positioned, we have the power today to unify and author a new story, together.

PART I:
HISTORICAL FOUNDATIONS OF DEHUMANIZATION

The myth of Black biological inferiority was not a historical accident. It emerged as a deliberate strategy, carefully constructed and systematically maintained, to justify the brutal enslavement of African people and safeguard the economic and social dominance of colonial elites. Early colonial leaders, faced with the threat of unity among oppressed laborers, recognized the need to create permanent divisions along racial lines. In response, a racial hierarchy was codified, establishing people of African descent as inherently different, dangerous, and subhuman. This fabricated narrative of inferiority was not only used to divide and conquer but also to rationalize the unthinkable: the transformation of human beings into property.

What made this system of oppression so enduring was the way physical and psychological barriers of dehumanization worked hand in hand, reinforcing one another to produce a self-perpetuating cycle of harm. The extreme physical exploitation of enslaved Africans—relentless labor, violence, and denial of basic human rights—was justified through assertions of biological deficiency. Meanwhile, the psychological torment of enslavement, the systematic stripping of identity, culture, autonomy, and dignity, served to reinforce the same narratives of inferiority. Together, these mechanisms upheld the institution of slavery and embedded a legacy of dehumanization so deep that it erected barriers to wellness for both the enslaved and their dependents.

The dehumanization of African people was further cemented by influential voices of the time: politicians, theologians, and particularly physicians and scientists actively promoting pseudoscientific theories claiming that people of African descent were biologically suited for enslavement. These falsehoods were disseminated through religious sermons, legal codes, medical texts, and educational institutions, creating a cultural ecosystem in which the abuse and neglect of Black bodies and minds could be both normalized and perpetuated. Part I of this book examines the foundational barriers of dehumanization through a historical lens, focusing on how physical and psychological harm converged to entrench the lie of

Black inferiority. This convergence established deep and lasting obstacles to health and well-being, barriers that have persisted across generations, shaping the wellness outcomes of African Americans long after the formal end of slavery.

CHAPTER 1:
THE MYTH OF INFERIORITY: THE ORIGIN STORY

To grapple with the concept of African Americans experiencing barriers to wellness, one must first understand the power of the narrative of biological inferiority. This living, breathing, moving concept became the primary driver behind a growing nation's acceptance of the dehumanization of enslaved Africans then and complicity in the impact it has on its descendants now. The American institution of slavery was more than an economic enterprise; it was a system that relied on deeply entrenched ideological constructs to maintain its operations. By the 19th century, slavery was an estimated 3.5 billion-dollar industry, equating to approximately $23 trillion today.[1]

To sustain such a profitable system, it was essential for American society to believe that people of African descent were inherently suited to bondage and labor. This belief helped to define Black individuals as biologically and morally inferior, a narrative that bolstered social acceptance of slavery and prevented challenges to its legitimacy. Without this pervasive belief, maintaining a system that deprived millions of people of their basic human rights would have been politically and morally unsustainable. That is the power of dehumanization; it tricks people into accepting behavior they would otherwise immediately recognize as unethical and unfair. Thus, a mythology of Black inferiority was created and promoted, painting people of African descent as less than human and emphasizing their "natural" fitness for servitude.

Social consensus on the concept of biological inferiority not only contradicts a natural tendency toward human compassion and allyship but also produces distinctions strong enough to justify barriers. These barriers determine who is on the side of access to resources, rights, and privileges and who is undeserving. Society at large accepted this ideology around white supremacy and Black inferiority. Therefore, as American society was emerging in its earliest form, Black inferiority was melded into its core like an egg into a fully baked cake. Regardless of the size of the slice or whether or not it has frosting, the concept of racial discrimination is inescapable. The only way to make the cake vegan, or in this case, more equitable and just for everyone to consume it without problems, is to bake a new cake. If only rebuilding a nation without racial discrimination were as easy as baking a cake. Until there is a collective reckoning with the historical abuses built from the aforementioned falsehoods and a deliberate effort to dismantle the structures they have created, Black individuals will continue to face barriers in achieving optimal health and well-being, making them more vulnerable to disease prevalence.

Rebellion and Control: The Aftermath of Bacon's Rebellion

Bacon's Rebellion of 1676 marked a critical turning point in the establishment of racial divisions within colonial America. This uprising, led by Nathaniel Bacon, brought together European and African laborers, both indentured and enslaved, who shared a common desire to challenge the colonial government's disregard for their grievances. Despite their differing origins, these disenfranchised groups united in resistance against oppressive labor conditions, the monopoly of land by the elite, and the lack of governmental protection. As historian Ibram X. Kendi observes, this rebellion represented a direct threat to Virginia landowners. For them, it meant, "that poor whites had to be forever separated from enslaved Blacks."[2]

In response, the colonial government acted decisively, instituting measures that would sever such cross-racial alliances and solidify a racial hierarchy that privileged whiteness, even among economically disadvantaged Europeans.

Prior to the rebellion, European indentured servants and enslaved Africans frequently interacted, working side by side and building bonds based on shared oppression. This commingling threatened the colonial elite, who feared that a united lower class could overthrow the existing power structures. Following the rebellion's suppression, colonial authorities implemented a strategy designed to divide and control the laboring class by embedding racial distinctions into the legal and social fabric of the colony. Jacqueline Battlora in *Birth of a Nation* points out how these changes "altered those relationships of mutuality, cooperation, and trust between persons of African and European ancestry."[3] Gaining patriarchal allies among poor Europeans was strategic and deliberate. As historian Edmund Morgan suggests, poor whites received a "fictive" elevation of status, rooted solely in their racial identity rather than any genuine economic improvement.[4] This hollow elevation replaced the promise of land or wealth with a socially constructed privilege based on whiteness, which became the basis of a new social hierarchy.

The colonial government moved swiftly to enforce such racial divisions through an array of legal measures and social controls, which served both to strip people of African descent of rights and to indoctrinate poor landless whites with a sense of racial superiority. Laws were enacted that restricted the full participation of Black people in society. They were barred from holding property or weapons, and their mobility within the colony was curtailed. These measures placed Black bodies under constant surveillance and subjected them to brutal enforcement mechanisms, such as slave patrols. Initially limited to slaveholders, slave patrol duties soon became compulsory for all white men, even those without property. This imbued white society with a sense of power and authority that

PART I: HISTORICAL FOUNDATIONS OF DEHUMANIZATION

was grounded solely in race, embedding a culture of racial policing into the daily lives of white citizens. Poor whites, who might otherwise have aligned with African laborers based on economic interests, were encouraged instead to view themselves as protectors of the racial order, responsible for policing the activities and movements of Black individuals. Kendi refers to the poor whites' new role as "the armed defenders of planters –a place that would sow bitter animosity between them and enslaved Africans."[5]

The creation of a legally enforced racial hierarchy ultimately reshaped Virginia's social landscape. As Battalora points out, "white laborers were given little more than the authority to rule over their fellow laborers of African descent and members of native tribes on the premise that they share a superior status with elites–whiteness."[6] This sense of racial unity provided poor whites with a psychological sense of empowerment, as the continuous stripping away of African rights affirmed their place above Black individuals within the social hierarchy. The elite successfully restructured Virginia society, binding poor whites to a racial identity that offered no material benefit but promised a sense of superiority over African Americans. The manufactured solidarity rooted in whiteness obscured the economic realities of poverty, creating a society that would remain divided along racial lines rather than united against the true sources of economic oppression.

Economic, social, and political fears appear very real in the eyes of the beholders, making them ripe for governmental control via manipulation. The aftermath of Bacon's Rebellion is only one example among others where the government manipulates "False Evidence to Appear as Real" (FEAR) as part of a strategy to maintain power. The use of skin tone to pit whites against Blacks simplified undeniable distinctions between the two groups.

Colonial Americans used skin tone to create identities through which to employ their divide and conquer strategy. What happens when two ethnic groups have an equivalent amount of melanin concentration, sharing genetics, culture, and linguistics, such as the Hutus and the Tutsis in Rwanda? Their social stratification was class-based: Hutus could work towards elevation of status, become chiefs, and evolve into Tutsis. This made ethnicity a fluid concept for them, that is, until the Belgian government came along and changed the narrative, paving a path towards the treachery of the Rwandan Genocide in 1994 that left hundreds of thousands of people brutally massacred over the course of 100 days.

The Rwandan genocide of 1994 definitely stands as a harsh illustration of how colonial legacies and state-sanctioned narratives can culminate in catastrophic violence. Leading up to these events was Belgian colonial rule and its impact on social dynamics. Physical features such as skulls, noses, and height were measured to place citizens into one fixed ethnic category, politically reinforced by the requirement to carry ethnic identity cards. Social mobility under colonial rule favored the Tutsi, with the institutionalized hierarchy sowing deep-seated resentment among the Hutu, who formed a majority. The privileges towards the Tutsis prevailed until the Hutu-led republic replaced their monarchy.

Post-independence, Hutu elites were determined to capitalize on ethnic divisions as a means to retain power. They employed state-sponsored media like Radio Télévision Libre des Mille Collines (RTLM) to disseminate hate speech, referring to Tutsis as "cockroaches" and inciting violence against them. One of the most blunt directives broadcast across the radio waves was the call to "cut down the tall trees," a euphemism urging the extermination of Tutsis.[7] These were not mere labels or words; it was the power of using dehumanizing speech to fuel and embolden the fear-based consciousness of everyday citizens, thereby manipulating them to murder their neighbors violently. This orchestrated dehumanization exemplifies how constructed identities and state-sanctioned narratives can mobilize populations toward violence, reinforcing the dangers of fear-based social divisions.

Both situations, the Rwandan Genocide and the aftermath of Bacon's Rebellion, demonstrate how colonial authorities fostered a

PART I: HISTORICAL FOUNDATIONS OF DEHUMANIZATION

racialized social order to manipulate social divisions and maintain their grip on power. The harrowing details of the Rwandan Genocide serve to ground us in the reality of the dangerous nature of racialized or ethnicity-based dehumanization. Many Americans take our racialized system for granted, a status quo, perhaps, but are more easily able to recognize similar systems as horrific when decontextualized from their own tradition of a racialized society.

In the American case, Black individuals were systematically excluded from the emerging narrative of American identity, positioned instead as a permanent underclass whose humanity was continuously denied. The long-term consequences of these practices created a dual narrative: one of privilege and belonging as whiteness and one of perpetual struggle and exclusion as Blackness. For the dominant culture, the arising American identity became one of freedom, opportunity, and advancement. But for Black individuals, it became an experience defined by oppression, dispossession, and survival. The colonial government's plan was so brilliantly executed that for hundreds of years, the social hierarchy, understanding, and acceptance remained in place and have not been challenged. Unfortunately, this social reality created profound psychological impacts on the Black community. Generations of African Americans have endured internalizing the experience of being treated as "other," as society develops more sophisticated mechanisms to suppress both their sense of freedom and self-worth.

This imposed identity, constructed through centuries of legal and social reinforcement, was more than just a societal narrative; it carried with it severe repercussions on all aspects of Black health and well-being. As research continues to reveal, the chronic stress associated with racism and social exclusion has profound biological and psychological effects, contributing to elevated risks of hypertension, metabolic disorders, and other adverse health outcomes within the Black community. Through laws and social practices that alienated Black individuals from humanity, American society established a system of racial toxicity and its associated barriers that continue to negatively shape both cultural identity and health outcomes today.

Thought Leaders of Oppression

Laws targeting Black Americans were only the beginning of a carefully constructed racist ideology to maintain a relatively unchallenged justification of economic, political, and social exploitation of people of African descent and their descendants. Reconditioning social behavior was not enough. There had to be a deep-seated shift in attitudes and belief systems that was unquestionably internalized, fully embraced, and embodied by the masses as the inherent truth. This indoctrination of a narrative of biological inferiority would not only become easy for white social acceptance, but it would also become a nearly inescapable message permeating the consciousness of many of the enslaved Africans and their descendants.

The high rollers of social influence used their ranks as intellectuals, physicians, scientists, and other public figures to propagate and widely disseminate the false narrative of Black inferiority. These influencers leveraged both their positions and platforms to give a credible voice to their unsubstantiated ideology. As noted by historian, Harriet Washington in *Medical Apartheid*, "the scientific racist's emphasis was not upon fact-based theories, logical methodologies, experimental data, control groups, and verification by replication."[8] By embedding these ideas into the emerging fields of medicine, anthropology, and biology, they provided the so-called "scientific evidence" needed to justify slavery, systemic racism, and the exclusion of African Americans from the full rights of citizenship. This "scientific evidence" gave elite society a pseudo-rational basis for regarding Black people as naturally inferior, reinforcing a social order that benefited from the continued exploitation of Black bodies from the cradle to the grave.

These ideologies continue to influence racial disparities and biases today, perpetuating sustained barriers in all aspects of life for many African Americans. These barriers that lead to poorer health outcomes came from the historical and contemporary navigation of what it means on a cellular level to live in a systemically oppressive environment. I will highlight five of the primary architects of this false narrative to examine how the nihilism around Black wellness first came about.

Charles Caldwell (1772-1853)

Physician and Promoter of Phrenology

Charles Caldwell, a prominent 19th-century American physician and educator, played a foundational role in embedding medical racism into early American scientific thought. Through his writings and academic influence, Caldwell helped justify the dehumanization of Black people under the guise of medical and scientific authority. As a staunch supporter of phrenology—a pseudoscience that claimed a person's intellect and character could be determined by skull shape—Caldwell spread phrenology-based theories on the biological inferiority of African-descended people. In his work *Thoughts on the Original Unity of the Human Race* (1852), Caldwell rejected the idea of racial equality, claiming that Africans were "constitutionally and intellectually" inferior to whites.[9] He argued that the cranial features of Black people revealed a natural predisposition for subservience and limited intellectual capacity, supporting the racist notion that slavery was a natural and appropriate condition for African Americans.

Caldwell also promoted the belief that Black people were physically different in ways that suited them for manual labor in hot climates.[10] As a professor at institutions like Transylvania University and what is now known as the University of Louisville, Caldwell taught and influenced generations of physicians. His racial theories were not fringe beliefs—they became part of the mainstream medical curriculum in the antebellum South. By embedding racial hierarchy into medical education, Caldwell helped institutionalize racist assumptions that would persist throughout American medical history. Overall, he used his scientific platform to validate slavery, devalue Black humanity, and normalize racial disparities in medicine. He paved the way for other influencers to extrapolate additional so-called "biological differences" that would further place the health of the Black population at risk. Comprehensively, these theories helped form the early medical myths that Black people had thicker skin, higher pain thresholds, and required less medical care—ideas that have been debunked but still contribute to present-day disparities in pain management and medical treatment. Caldwell's legacy is a stark example of how pseudoscience and racial ideology worked hand-in-hand to shape systemic bias in healthcare—biases that continue to affect the health and well-being of African Americans today.

Samuel Cartwright (1793-1863)

Physician and Proponent of "Scientific Racism"

Samuel A. Cartwright was a physician who became nationally recognized not only as a medical authority but also as an ethnologist and racial theorist. Based in the antebellum South, he is widely known as one of the most notorious figures in the history of American medical racism. His work exemplifies how pseudoscience was used to legitimize slavery and reinforce the belief in Black inferiority, embedding racist ideologies into the foundations of American medicine. Cartwright gained infamy for inventing and promoting fictitious medical diagnoses under an umbrella of what Washington refers to as "Black Diseases," where he pathologized the behavior of enslaved Blacks.[11] Most notably, he coined the condition "Drapetomania" in 1851, which he described as a mental illness that caused enslaved people to flee captivity.[12] Rather than acknowledging the obvious human desire for freedom, Cartwright framed escape as a symptom of disease, suggesting that slavery was the natural and healthy condition for Black people. Pathologizing normal human behavior, specifically the desire for freedom, served to reinforce stereotypes of Black intellectual inferiority and laziness, giving medical backing to white supremacist beliefs. To further throw salt in the wound, he even proposed that "treatments" for drapetomania include whipping and the enforcement of strict labor discipline.

Also, under his "Black Diseases" line, Cartwright created another pseudoscientific diagnosis, which he termed Cachexia Africana, a label for the tendency of some of the enslaved to consume non-nutritive substances such as clay, chalk, or dirt—a mental health condition presently recognized as pica (not race specified). However, people who demonstrate signs of pica often have mineral deficiencies, such as calcium or iron, which was typical amongst the enslaved population. Rather than interpreting this behavior as a symptom of chronic malnutrition, Cartwright naturally viewed it as further evidence of racial degeneracy. His work illustrates how medicine was weaponized to normalize oppression, transforming survival responses into evidence of inferiority and turning the enslaved body into a site of state-sanctioned pathology. As demonstrated by historian Todd Savitt, Cartwright's work extended beyond the medical sector and into "the political realm to justify the white southern point of view."[13] These so-called diagnoses ignored the brutal reality of life under slavery, where nutritional deprivation, physical abuse, and psychological trauma were routine. In medicalizing the effects of such substandard living conditions, Cartwright did more than distort science—he dehumanized an entire population to protect the institution of slavery.

Cartwright's work became widespread as he leveraged his position as a member of the Medical Association of Louisiana and a contributor to the *New Orleans Medical and Surgical Journal* to disseminate his theories across multiple platforms. His writings were circulated among Southern physicians, planters, and policymakers, and they were used to justify both the continuation of slavery and the unequal treatment of Black patients within the medical system. Furthermore, Cartwright's work exemplified how race-based science became a tool of social control. By disguising racial prejudice as medical knowledge, Cartwright, as described by historian Peter Kolchin, attempted to demonstrate "that Blacks were by nature different, inferior, and thereby unsuited for freedom."[14] These ideas would echo into the post-emancipation era, shaping public health policies and justifying the medical neglect of African Americans into the 21st century.

Samuel Morton (1799-1851)
Physician, Anthropologist, and Founder of Craniometry

Samuel George Morton, a Philadelphia-based physician and natural scientist, played a central role in developing and legitimizing scientific racism in 19th-century America. His work on craniometry—the measurement of skulls—was presented as objective science, but, in reality, it provided a powerful pseudo-scientific foundation for beliefs in Black inferiority and the supposed natural racial hierarchy.

Morton collected and measured hundreds of human skulls from around the world, publishing his findings in works such as *Crania Americana* (1839) and *Crania Aegyptiaca* (1844). He claimed that cranial capacity could determine intellectual ability and that different races had inherently different brain sizes. According to his measurements, Morton concluded that Europeans had the largest skulls and thus the highest intellectual capacities, while Africans had the smallest skulls, which he interpreted as proof of lesser intelligence.[15]

As the Father of Anthropology, Morton won worldwide respect as the world's premier empiricist on racial typology and ethnology questions."[16] Although he portrayed his work as unbiased and empirical, modern analysis reveals that his conclusions were deeply influenced by racial bias. Anthropologist Stephen Jay Gould famously reanalyzed Morton's data in *The Mismeasure of Man* (1981), arguing that Morton manipulated methods and selectively reported results to align with his belief in white superiority.[17] While some scholars have debated aspects of Gould's critique, there remains widespread consensus that Morton's work reinforced racial hierarchies under the guise of scientific legitimacy.

Morton's racial typology placed Africans at the bottom of the intellectual and moral spectrum. His work was used to support polygenism—the theory that different races were created separately and were biologically distinct. This theory stood in contrast to monogenism, which held that all humans shared a common origin. By advocating for the biological separateness and inferiority of Black people, Morton's findings were eagerly embraced by pro-slavery advocates and medical professionals in the South, who cited his work as scientific justification for the subjugation and mistreatment of African-descended populations.[18]

Morton's legacy is a clear example of how flawed scientific practices were used to reinforce social and political ideologies. His work provided intellectual ammunition for medical racism by helping to entrench the belief that Black people were inherently less intelligent, more primitive, and biologically different—assumptions that influenced not only slavery-era medicine but also medical education and healthcare disparities well into the 20th century.

Josiah Nott (1804-1873)

Surgeon, Anthropologist, and Co-Author of Types of Mankind

Josiah Clark Nott, a Southern physician and anthropologist from Alabama, was a central figure in the entrenchment of medical and scientific racism in 19th-century America. His work was heavily influenced by polygenism, thereby providing a powerful intellectual framework for justifying slavery, racial segregation, and the belief in Black biological inferiority. As a student of the previously mentioned Samuel George Morton and a staunch supporter of his craniometric theories, Nott expanded upon Morton's work by blending pseudoscience with pro-slavery ideology. In his widely circulated writings, including *Types of Mankind* (1854), co-authored with George Gliddon, Nott argued that Black people were a separate and inferior species to whites.[19] Knott argued that polygenesis was a part of the natural order. His book became the single text most responsible for setting the issue of race in a scientific context for the general public."[20] Therefore, helping to solidify into the consciousness of society that African-descended people were physically and mentally suited only for servitude.[21] Nott's theories were deeply racialized and often cloaked in the language of scientific objectivity. He rejected monogenist views and claimed that the Bible supported polygenism, thus trying to reconcile his scientific racism with Christian theology. By doing so, he appealed to both Southern slaveholders and religious audiences who were looking for both moral and intellectual justification for the continued enslavement of African Americans.[22]

Perhaps most troubling of all, Nott explicitly linked race to disease and health. He claimed that Black people were constitutionally different from whites and required different medical treatment, a belief that fueled disparities in care and laid early groundwork for racially segregated medicine. For example, he theorized that diseases like yellow fever and malaria affected Black and white bodies differently, implying an inherent biological difference in susceptibility and immunity.[23] This bolstered the myth that Black people were biologically suited for labor in hot, disease-prone climates, again serving the interests of Southern plantation economies at the expense of Black health and wellness.

Lastly, Josiah Nott used his lectures, publications, and medical practice to gain far-reaching impact. His contributions to medical racism were grounded in his efforts to fuse pseudoscientific racial theory with medical thought. He helped popularize the idea that scientific evidence proved Black inferiority and validated racial hierarchies.[24] These ideas were not only socially corrosive but also had lasting effects on medical education and treatment standards, reinforcing systemic bias in healthcare for generations. His advocacy for polygenism, support of slavery, and promotion of race-based medicine contributed significantly to the structural racism that has shaped American medicine and whose effects remain evident in contemporary health disparities.

James Marion Sims (1813-1883)

Physician, "Father of Modern Gynecology."

James Marion Sims, often referred to as the "father of modern gynecology," occupies a deeply controversial place in medical his-

PART I: HISTORICAL FOUNDATIONS OF DEHUMANIZATION

tory. While he is credited with surgical advancements in women's reproductive health, particularly the treatment of vesicovaginal fistulas, his legacy is inseparable from the medical racism and exploitation that enabled his work. Sims conducted invasive, painful, and repeated gynecological surgeries on enslaved Black women without anesthesia or consent, practices that exemplify the brutal intersection of racism, medicine, and slavery in the 19th century.

Between 1845 and 1849, Sims experimented on at least eleven enslaved women in Alabama, including three women whose names are known: Anarcha, Betsey, and Lucy. These women were subjected to multiple surgeries, often without any form of anesthesia, under the racist belief that Black people, especially Black women, did not feel pain the same way white people did. Sims' justifications reflected the broader pseudoscientific narrative of the time: that Black bodies were biologically different and could endure more suffering.[25] Sims never obtained consent from these women, nor did he regard them as patients with rights. Instead, they were seen as medical property whose suffering was acceptable for the advancement of white women's reproductive health. The fact that his earliest surgical successes came at the expense of these Black women reveals how the American medical establishment was built, in part, on the exploitation of the enslaved.

Despite his unethical methods, Sims gained acclaim and institutional recognition. He later founded the first women's hospital in the U.S., served as president of the American Medical Association, and was celebrated by the medical profession for more than a century. Statues of Sims were erected in multiple cities, often without acknowledgment of the human cost of his research. It wasn't until recent years, amid increased attention to systemic racism in medicine, that public and scholarly voices began to critically reassess his legacy, leading to the removal of his statue in New York City in 2018.

Sims' work has had a lasting impact on the trust Black communities place in the healthcare system. His experiments epitomize the historical exploitation of Black bodies in the name of scientific progress and contribute to a generational trauma that continues to affect how Black patients, particularly Black women, experience and access medical care today. His medical contributions cannot be separated from the racialized violence and ethical violations at their core. Marion Sims' legacy is definitely a stark reminder that the foundations of modern medicine are entangled with slavery and racism. Furthermore, it supports the case for reckoning with this history in order to confront present-day health inequities.

Pseudoscience Shaping Contemporary Health

The pseudo-scientific theories of Caldwell, Morton, Cartwright, Nott, and Sims assisted in laying the intellectual and institutional foundation for racial bias in American medicine. This legacy remains evident in healthcare disparities experienced by African Americans today. These men promoted deeply harmful beliefs: that Black people were biologically inferior, more tolerant of pain, mentally less capable, and constitutionally suited for labor and disease. While modern medicine has advanced beyond the blatant pseudoscience of the 19th century, the implicit biases seeded by these thinkers continue to show up in provider behavior, patient outcomes, and systemic inequities.

One of the most enduring myths with roots in this legacy is the false belief that Black people have higher pain thresholds. James Marion Sims and Samuel Cartwright promoted the idea that Black individuals could endure extreme physical suffering without the need for anesthesia or comfort. Today, this myth is echoed in studies showing that Black patients are significantly less likely to receive adequate pain medication compared to white patients, even when presenting with the same conditions.[26] This disconnect in pain management affects emergency room care, postoperative recovery, and the treatment of chronic pain, and it fosters mistrust between patients and providers. All of which feeds into a cycle of increasing health disparities in the African American population.

Likewise, the work of Samuel Morton and Josiah Nott, who framed Black people as intellectually inferior and biologically distinct, helped cement a legacy of differential treatment in diagnostic and clinical settings. Modern examples include the use of race-based corrections in algorithms for kidney function (eGFR), lung capacity, and heart failure risk—tools that adjust results downward for Black patients, often delaying diagnosis or access to treatment.[27] These practices are slowly being reevaluated, but they remain embedded in the software, protocols, and habits of many healthcare systems.

Charles Caldwell and Cartwright's assertions about the "natural suitability" of Black people for servitude and their supposed insensitivity to disease have modern echoes in how African Americans are often deprioritized or dismissed during routine healthcare interactions. African American women, for example, are more likely to have their symptoms minimized or ignored during childbirth, contributing to a maternal mortality rate nearly three times higher than that of white women.[28] This is particularly alarming given that these outcomes persist across income and education levels, demonstrating that racism, not class, drives the disparity.

Ultimately, the legacy of these 19th-century figures endures not because their science was sound, but because of their positions in society as thought leaders. Their racist ideas were woven into the fabric of medical institutions, hence the enduring legacy of their ideologies. This legacy is evident in today's clinical guidelines, provider education, and even in interpersonal assumptions. For African Americans, this means navigating a healthcare system where distrust is often rational and where advocacy is not just self-care but survival. Unraveling the damage requires more than reform; it calls for a critical reckoning with medicine's racist past and its present-day consequences.

America's Enduring Image of Blackness

The American public, century after century, has been socially conditioned to accept and even defend systems that harm Black bodies. This psychological programming, first seeded during the colonial era with the institutionalization of race following Bacon's Rebellion, was cultivated through law, policy, medicine, education, and media. Thought leaders, medical professionals, and public officials served as the architects of a dangerous illusion, one that justified the degradation of African-descended people to maintain the status quo. That illusion has morphed over time but never disappeared. Instead, it rebrands itself in new forms that appear as mass incarceration, redlining, environmental injustice, under-resourced healthcare, and biased clinical practices.

When we look closely, America is not just looking at Black suffering; it is looking at itself. The disproportionate rates of hypertension, diabetes, maternal mortality, and mental illness in Black communities do not originate in biology; they are reflections of historical trauma, structural abuse, and long-standing national neglect. Each diagnosis, each preventable death, is not only a public health failure but also a moral one. Yet and still, the nation continues to treat these outcomes as disconnected, individualized tragedies rather than interconnected symptoms of historical systemic design. America has employed a centuries-long apparatus of denial, one that allows the majority to look away, to disassociate, or worse, to justify the suffering they see. Society is blind to the cause of disease vulnerabilities within the Black community while judging the community for having the audacity to be vulnerable and not doing anything about it ourselves.

But mirrors, even when distorted, do not lie. They may bend the truth, but the truth remains visible for those who choose to see. Furthermore, what is reflected back at us is not just the enduring harm done to African Americans, but the deep moral compromise of a nation built on contradiction: liberty for some and "pseudo" freedom for others; healing for some and harm for others; acceptance for some and rejection for others. The visible outcomes of disease, disfigurement, and despair are the grotesque consequences of a story never truly reconciled. Until the nation collectively acknowledges this reflection and takes responsibility for what is staring back, the

PART I: HISTORICAL FOUNDATIONS OF DEHUMANIZATION

illusion will remain intact, fragile, fractured, yet tragically believable. Only through confronting the truth, unfiltered and unmasked, can America begin to shatter the falsehoods that have long defined its identity and dare to construct a new, more equitable reality.

Conclusion

As we close this chapter, it is important to recognize that the narrative of biological inferiority and its devastating consequences did not emerge in isolation; it was born from a carefully constructed system designed to justify exploitation and erase the humanity of African Americans. The calculated dehumanization of African-descended people laid a foundation for both social and medical discrimination that still shapes the experiences of African Americans today. What began as a political strategy evolved into a generational inheritance of trauma, misrepresentation, and systemic neglect. Yet, even in the face of centuries of distortion, erasure, and harm, the truth of our ancestors' resilience continues to rise. It reminds us that our collective healing must begin with collective remembering, remembering not only the suffering but also the survival, not just the oppression but also the overcoming.

The chapters ahead invite us to sit with the uncomfortable truths of our past, not to dwell in pain, but to honor the lived realities of those who endured enslavement and all its horrors. Their stories are not just historical artifacts; they are mirrors reflecting how deeply rooted inequities became embedded in the structures we navigate today. These truths deserve more than a footnote; they demand our full attention. Let this journey through history deepen our compassion, awaken our understanding, and fuel a greater commitment to dismantling the false ideologies that continue to cause harm. Because our ancestors endured more than we can imagine, we owe them the dignity of remembrance, the courage of truth-telling, and the responsibility of change.

CHAPTER 2:
EMBODIED EXPLOITATION: THE PHYSICAL TOLL OF SLAVERY ON BLACK HEALTH

In its 1946 preamble, the World Health Organization (WHO) defines health as "a state of complete physical, mental, and social well-being, and not merely the absence of disease or infirmity."[29] By this standard, neither enslaved Africans in the United States nor their descendants have ever experienced true health since their forced migration beginning in 1619. The institution of slavery systematically stripped enslaved Africans of their physical, emotional, and social well-being, creating conditions that perpetuated suffering, disease, and heightened health vulnerabilities for generations to come. Everything we know about the trans-Atlantic Slave trade would be contraindicated in the health and well-being of any group of people, regardless of race, ethnicity, or geography.

The daily reality of dehumanization experienced from the point of captivity and onward by enslaved Africans fostered an environment where disease was not only prevalent but almost inevitable. Overcrowded living quarters, poor sanitation, inadequate nutrition, and relentless physical labor created a breeding ground for illness. Yet, the damage extended far beyond the physical. Enslaved Africans endured constant psychological assaults designed to break their spirits and suppress resistance, stripping them of autonomy,

PART I: HISTORICAL FOUNDATIONS OF DEHUMANIZATION

community, and dignity. Their identities were fractured under the weight of systemic violence, leaving scars that would ripple across generations. The consequences of this brutal system were reflected in life expectancy statistics. While white Americans in the 19th century often lived to 40-43 years of age, the average lifespan of an enslaved Black person was just 21-22 years, less than half of their white counterparts.[30] These disparities were not random but the direct result of an existence defined by exploitation, deprivation, and relentless torment. Slavery was not only a socioeconomic institution but also a system that weaponized health and well-being as tools of oppression.

As we dive into this exploration of historical dehumanization, we must consider the profound impact of these lived realities. The health outcomes experienced by enslaved Africans and their descendants were calculated byproducts of a system that prioritized wealth over humanity. These conditions created a legacy of cellular trauma that is still evident in the health disparities faced by African Americans today. Understanding this history is essential to unpacking the roots of racial toxicity and the wellness barriers it built.

Cape Coast Reflection

A day that began with great wonder, curiosity, and excitement for me concluded with gut-wrenching pain and grief while visiting the Cape Coast of Ghana, West Africa, in November of 2023. It was there that I, along with a small group of friends, was met by the local grounds tour guide, who recounted the history of our ancestors' journey into enslavement. We were told that after being violently seized from their respective villages or sold into captivity by other natives, countless Africans were then forcibly marched for days or weeks to coastal trading posts. This march was far unlike that of the military regime or any HBCU marching band; it was void of pride, dignity, and even humanity. Depending on the location in which they were captured, some enslaved Africans would take over two million steps (the equivalent of 1000 miles) across rugged terrain while shackled together in chains under the kiss of a fierce sunlight radiating oppres-

sive heat. For them, this trek was far beyond physically grueling, as approximately half would lose their lives as they succumbed to the exhaustion, hunger, and injuries they suffered along the way. An ill fate also fell upon those who struggled to keep up with the majority, whereas they were often beaten or killed on the spot, leaving a trail of human remains. The survival of the fittest would eventually make it to what is known today as the Assin Manso Slave River Site, where we were now being told their story. My group and I had adorned ourselves in all-white attire as a part of our ancestral veneration. There we stood in the river singing Old Negro Spirituals while reenacting the "Last Bath" they would ever have on African soil. Little did we know, the visceral reactions we were experiencing in that moment were about to be amplified 24 miles up the road at the Cape Coast Castle, which was our next stop and also their final holding place before their forced migration into the Americas, the Caribbean, and South America.

Unlike other tours at this site that took place during the day, so we were told, our personal trip tour guide arranged for our group to visit the dungeons at night for a more immersive experience, and that we had, indeed. With lit candles, open ears, and bright, wide eyes too scared to blink, we carefully crossed the cruel dungeon floor. Cold and heartless concrete that once held the bare-skinned bodies of our chained ancestors as they lay crammed together with no reprieve from the sweltering heat of bodies upon bodies commingling in one another's vomit, sweat, urine, feces, and menstrual blood. Some aspects of this part of the tour guide's narration were not new information to me, but the moment he mentioned "menstrual blood," it was another layer of this horrendous violence I had not heard mentioned until that very moment, nor had I ever stopped to consider it, and it triggered something inside of me beyond not only being a person of African ancestry, but as a doctor who is also a woman. The thought of women being forced to lie in the free flow of not only their own menstrual blood but also that of hundreds of other women that surrounded them was downright repulsive to me.

PART I: HISTORICAL FOUNDATIONS OF DEHUMANIZATION

There I stood on this dungeon floor that was once soaked with evidence of human cruelty inflicted upon people who belonged to their immediate families, their communities. They were husbands, wives, mothers, fathers, sons, daughters, brothers, sisters, aunts, uncles, nieces, nephews, and cousins now missing, missing forever, never to be heard from, seen, or touched by their loved ones again. The heart-wrenching grief of that alone is enough to cause anyone to drown in an undeniable ocean of sorrow. Yet and still, compounded treachery ensued with every inhale they took of the vile stench and unavoidable exposure to cross-contamination with a concrete cesspool of bacteria.

The brutality of the dungeon became a breeding ground for not only physical disease but also the mental and emotional anguish this tomb of despair triggered. As horrendous as the dungeon experience was for our ancestors, it would only be just the initial layer of their multi-tiered journey of torture as they prepared to cross the threshold of the "Door of No Return." Once they were herded like cattle aboard the ships and stowed below deck as human cargo sailing the Atlantic sea, they would never be greeted with the love, kindness, compassion, and respect of kin; they had once known only to be left with sheer memories. They would also never experience the rich culture and customs that shaped their identity. They would never see their homeland of Mother Africa again.

The Middle Passage

The large ships transporting enslaved Africans were deliberately overloaded to maximize profits while simultaneously perpetuating a floating hub of disease. Cruelty continued and perhaps even heightened as the enslaved were brutally introduced to the vastness of the Atlantic Ocean, which many had never seen before. The infamous British ship Brookes, documented in an 18th-century engraving, was designed to carry 454 individuals but often transported over 600, cramming men, women, and children into a cargo hold with as little as 4–6 square feet of space per person and approximately 3 feet high.[31] These conditions made it impossible for them to change positions, stretch, or stand erect except for when they were allowed on deck for daily exercise or dance. This voyage of torture to human bodies that are designed for some type of movement at least every 30 minutes was severely constricted to mostly stillness for a 5000-mile voyage that could take as long as six months, depending on weather conditions.

The motion of the ocean provoked seasickness on an already overcrowded ship of two-legged cargo restricted from movement at all, much less towards any hollowed-out containers to relieve themselves of bacteria-filled human excrements. Once again, they were left without a choice but to release it all on the wicked floor. Such accumulation created a stench so overwhelming that historians report that it could be detected miles away. Infectious diseases like dysentery, smallpox, and typhoid fever were among those that were spread throughout the ship. A firsthand account of the deplorable nature of this experience was depicted in an autobiography by Equiano, an African youth taken into captivity who eventually purchased his own freedom while in America. He reflects on being herded onto the ship:

> But this disappointment was the least of my sorrow. The stench of the hold while we were on the coast was so intolerably loathsome, that it was dangerous to remain there for any time, and some of us had been permitted to stay on the deck for the fresh air; but now that the whole ship's cargo were confined together, it became absolutely pestilential. The closeness of the place, and the heat of the climate, added to the number in the ship, which was so crowded that each had scarcely room to turn himself, almost suffocating us. This produced copious perspirations, so that the air soon became unfit for respiration, from a variety of loathsome smells, and brought on a sickness among the slaves, of which many died -- thus falling victims to the improvident avarice, as I may call it, of their purchasers. This wretched situation was again aggravated by the gaffing of the chains, now became insupportable.[32]

PART I: HISTORICAL FOUNDATIONS OF DEHUMANIZATION   43

Throughout the voyage, the continual suffocation of fresh air soon provoked the enchanting idea of death to Equiano, as he explains here:

"I was soon put down under the decks, and there I received such a salutation in my nostrils as I had never experienced in my life: so that, with the loathsomeness of the stench, and crying together, I became so sick and low that I was not able to eat, nor had I the least desire to taste anything. I now wished for the last friend, death, to relieve me; but soon, to my grief, two of the white men offered me eatables; and, on my refusing to eat, one of them held me fast by the hands, and laid me across, I think, the windlass, and tied my feet, while the other flogged me severely. I had never experienced anything of this kind before, and, although not being used to the water, I naturally feared that element the first time I saw it, yet, nevertheless, could I have got over the nettings, I would have jumped over the side, but I could not."[33]

Living death became a reality for the enslaved as they were dehydrated and starved with mere scraps of rice, beans, or yams, lacking sufficient nutritional intake, causing their bodies to grow weaker throughout the journey. Women and children—vulnerable in ways that defy words—were often targeted by the crew for sexual violence. As noted by Equiano, *"The shrieks of the women, and the groans of the dying, rendered the whole a scene of horror almost inconceivable."*[34] Unlike Equiano, many were able to seize the opportunity to create a different outcome for themselves despite the pain and agony of such a terrifying experience. Some did attempt suicide, and if caught, were flogged unmercifully for daring to prefer death over captivity. Then some found solace in the ocean's depths, after choosing to leap into the unknown rather than endure the torment of slavery any longer. There were also the courageous captives who dared to resist their captors by revolting; of which 55 detailed accounts were recorded between 1699 and 1845."[35] These acts of heroism to be let free or die trying unfortunately brought them face-to-face with savage punishments meant to break their will: beatings, whippings, and executions were carried out with calculated brutality.

From 1619 through 1808, when the slave trade was abolished, an estimated 12-15% of enslaved Africans perished during the voyage of the Middle Passage that carried approximately 12 million people. This translates to 1.2 to 1.8 million violent deaths. Deaths due to disease, malnutrition, punishment, and suicide together contributed to the staggering mortality rates aboard the slave ships. Readers, if you have not already, take a moment and just breathe.

As horrendous as this sounds and actually is, this initial historic recount of the Trans-Atlantic Slave Trade demands being examined through the lens of the narrative of biological inferiority imposed upon African Americans. The level of physical, mental, emotional, and spiritual torment endured by enslaved Africans who survived the Middle Passage is nothing short of miraculous. The diverse pool of Black Americans began with African ancestors brought over on disease-infested ships. Africans who demonstrated great spirit, great strength, great adaptability, great resilience, and an incredible will to survive. What exactly is inferior about that?

The majority of those held captive across the Atlantic Ocean survived the abuse, the cruelty, the rampant spread of disease and despair while aboard the ship, which was only the BEGINNING of their need to endure life on all six cylinders of navigating survival for centuries across dehumanizing and oppressive terrain. Facing barrier after barrier spanning across generations, barriers that could have easily led to the racial annihilation of African Americans. Yet and still, as a race of people, here we are still standing, still surviving because of the DNA of the original stock. Is biological inferiority the new term for "powerful?"

Unfortunately, the horrors of the Middle Passage were just the entry point, a grim prelude to a life of relentless trauma and dehumanization for enslaved Africans on American shores. Upon arrival in the Americas, they were confronted with a brutal reality marked by unrelenting labor, physical exploitation, and systemic viciousness. The plantations where they were forced to toil became sites of both economic production and unimaginable suffering, with the demands of their labor exacting a severe toll on their bodies. What science is only recently becoming aware of is the genetic imprint these brutalities have left on present-day African Americans (to be discussed more in Chapter 5).

Enslaved Labor as Health Suppression

The labor imposed upon enslaved Africans in the United States was nothing short of inhumane. From sunrise to sunset, six days a week—or, depending on the plantation owner, all seven—the enslaved worked under the watchful and often violent supervision of their oppressors. As told by formerly enslaved Laura Thornton, "You'd be in the field to work way before day and then work way into the night."[36] Historian Edward E. Baptist discusses how the enslaved labored under a system where torture and violence were not deviations but integral mechanisms for increasing productivity, particularly with daily cotton quotas. He writes, "enslavers used torture to exert continuous pressure on all hands to find ways to split the self and become disembodied as a left hand at work. This was why many planters and overseers whipped even —or perhaps especially—their fastest pickers."[37] This added insult to injury, as every ounce of productivity and beyond was squeezed from their grueling, physically demanding, and unending labor, with no regard for human limitations. Toiling in the cotton, sugar, and tobacco fields was backbreaking and monotonous.

The relentless nature of this labor had devastating consequences for physical health. Prolonged and strenuous activity caused overworked muscles to hypertrophy, while the repetitive motions of planting, harvesting, and transporting crops exacerbated joint stress, leading to early-onset arthritis and degenerative joint diseases.[38] Archaeological studies of skeletal remains from enslaved populations reveal significant evidence of musculoskeletal stress markers and premature wear on joints, consistent with physically abusive labor patterns. Malnutrition compounded these issues, weakening bones and impairing the body's ability to recover from exertion. Unlike free laborers who might restore their bodies with nutritious meals, restful sleep, and time off, the enslaved population was routinely denied these necessities. As described by Frederick Douglass (1845) as he recounts that, "There were no beds given the slaves, unless one coarse blanket be considered such... they find less difficulty from the want of beds, than from the want of time to sleep."[39] There were simply not enough hours in the day to work the fields and prepare their livelihood after work for continued work the next day, which left them in perpetual exhaustion.

Enslaved Blacks who worked beyond the fields fared no better. Harriet Jacobs recalls that her enslaver, "often took an inspection of the house, to see that no one was idle."[40] Meanwhile, those in skilled trades such as carpentry, blacksmithing, or domestic service also endured physically taxing conditions, often without appropriate tools or safeguards. Women, in particular, bore a double burden, laboring in the fields while fulfilling domestic roles within the plantation, all while facing the added physical toll of pregnancy and childbirth. Historian Deborah Gray White describes this as a uniquely brutal reality, writing that, "once slaveholders realized that the reproductive function of the female slave could yield a profit, the manipulation of procreative sexual relations became an integral part of the sexual exploitation of female slaves."[41] Their dual labor was extracted without regard for recovery, health, or human limits, reinforcing the commodification of Black bodies as mere instruments of production for the plantation in addition to breeding more hands to work on the plantations.

The psychological toll of these labor conditions cannot be overstated. Enslaved people were forced to suppress pain, exhaustion, and even severe injury to avoid punishment. Chronic stress, compounded by constant surveillance from the planters and overseers and accompanied by physical violence to keep them on task, created an environment of sustained physical and psychological trauma. More contemporary research indicates that this form of unrelenting stress leads to what is now recognized as toxic stress, a condition that disrupts bodily systems and increases vulnerability to chronic disease[42] (Discussed in Chapter 4). All of which likely

PART I: HISTORICAL FOUNDATIONS OF DEHUMANIZATION

contributed to a cycle of suffering that further weakened their ability to resist or recover.

In a society where a person's worth was measured solely by their productivity, the health of the enslaved was expendable. Plantation owners viewed illness and injury not as tragedies but as economic inconveniences, particularly during harvest season. As explained by historian Sharla Fett, "Such precautions (of health) gave way under the pressures of harvest or planting seasons when planters risked the fatigue, injury, and sickness of enslaved workers against the gathering or sowing of crops."[43] Consequently, the enslaved population was often forced to continue working despite any debilitating conditions. Those who could no longer meet the demands of labor due to illness or aging were frequently discarded, sold, subjected to medical experimentation, or left to die without care.

This brutal labor system, designed to maximize profit at any human cost, left a legacy of physical and psychological trauma. Its effects are still visible today in the health disparities experienced by African Americans. Chronic pain, musculoskeletal disorders, and nutritional deficiencies, common among enslaved populations, laid the foundation for generational health disparities. Current research links these historical traumas to ongoing racial health inequities, with African Americans experiencing higher rates of arthritis, metabolic disease, and stress-related conditions.[44] The shadow of slavery's inhumane labor conditions continues to shape the health outcomes of Black communities, underscoring the enduring impact of racialized exploitation.

Despite the grueling and inhumane labor conditions that defined plantation life, the enslaved population displayed remarkable resilience in both subtle and powerful ways. In the fields, enslaved Africans relied heavily on collective work songs—spirituals, call-and-response chants, and rhythmic field hollers—as a vital tool for survival and resistance. These songs served multiple purposes: they helped synchronize physical movements during grueling labor, provided emotional and psychological relief, and created a shared sense of identity and solidarity. The call-and-response structure, deeply rooted in West African musical traditions, not only reinforced communal bonds but also allowed enslaved individuals to communicate with one another in coded language. Spirituals, often infused with biblical themes of deliverance and suffering, carried layered meanings that white overseers could not always decipher. Beneath these religious overtones were hidden messages, directions for escape, warnings of danger, or subtle forms of resistance that affirmed agency and resilience. Singing together in the fields allowed enslaved Africans to maintain cultural memory, preserve oral history, and resist dehumanization. These musical expressions functioned as both a survival strategy and a form of defiance, enabling them to retain a sense of dignity and hope amid the brutal conditions of plantation life.

Dwellings of Disease

The living quarters of the enslaved were a profound reflection of their dehumanization, offering minimal shelter and appalling conditions that compounded both the physical and psychological toll of their existence. These poorly constructed shacks, made from rough-hewn wood, mud, or other substandard materials, barely shielded inhabitants from the elements. Cracks in the walls allowed cold winds to whip through during the winter months, and the roofs often leaked during rainstorms, leaving interiors damp and fostering mold growth. In the sweltering heat of summer, these small, cramped spaces became suffocating ovens, with no windows or ventilation to provide relief. As historian Peter Kolchin describes, the housing for enslaved Blacks was "crude but functional" during the antebellum period, a small step up from colonial times when they were forced to sleep in "barns, sheds, lofts, or, weather permitting, outdoors."[45] Insufficient habitation underscored the blatant disregard for their well-being, as described by formerly enslaved Rachel Adams with her own firsthand account. "Us lived in mud-daubed log cabins that had old stack chimblies made out of sticks and mud. Our old homemade beds didn't have no slats or metal springs neither. Dey used stout cords for springs. De cloth what dey made the ticks of dem old hay mattresses and pillos out of so coarse dat it scratched us little chillum most to death, it seemed lak to us dem days."[46]

Inside these quarters, the conditions were equally deplorable. Floors were typically made of packed dirt or rough wooden planks, while bedding consisted of makeshift pallets assembled from straw or discarded rags, offering minimal protection against the hard ground.[47] After long, punishing hours of labor in the fields, the enslaved returned to these meager shelters without the means to properly rest and recover. The absence of adequate sleep and restorative conditions worsened existing physical injuries, particularly those caused by repetitive strain and overexertion, ultimately exacerbating musculoskeletal disorders such as arthritis and degenerative joint disease.

Congestion intensified these hardships. As many as five to ten people were crammed into small, 1-2 room cabins, with barely enough space for a fraction of that number. Historian Todd Savitt (2002) points out that "overcrowding and unsanitary living conditions caused an increased incidence of respiratory diseases."[48] With stagnant air, no ventilation, and constant exposure to bodily waste and sickness, infectious diseases like tuberculosis, pneumonia, and influenza spread rapidly, especially during colder, damp seasons. Byrd & Clayton (2000) depict an uninhabitable living space for respectable human beings as they stated, "… most slave quarters were filthy, allowing huge pest and parasitic infestations and promoting disease associated with poor hygiene at the personal and environmental levels."[49] Enslaved individuals were often forced to wash in nearby streams when possible, or not at all; therefore, activities like bathing, hair washing, and haircuts were not a part of routine care. When combined with unwashed clothes and unclean beds, they were more susceptible to skin infections, lice, and various pest infestations. The lack of clean water and proper sanitation turned minor infections into deadly threats that further compromised their health, increasing vulnerability to illness and compounding the physical wear and tear caused by forced labor.

The absence of proper clothing also exacerbated the suffering endured within these quarters. Enslaved men, women, and children were typically issued, depending on the plantation, 1-4 single sets of coarse, ill-fitting garments made from cheap materials. These clothes, wholly inadequate for the rigors of plantation labor and seasonal weather extremes, quickly became soiled and tattered. Thin fabrics provided little defense against the winter cold or summer heat, leaving individuals exposed to sunburn, hypothermia, and injury. They were given shoes that did not properly fit, making going barefoot a more preferred option among the enslaved, thereby increasing the risk of tetanus exposure. Over time, the combination of poor clothing and harsh conditions further deteriorated their health, contributing to chronic illnesses and heightened susceptibility to infections.

The psychological toll of these living conditions was equally profound. While a home is meant to offer safety, dignity, and rest, the quarters of the enslaved offered none of these. Instead, they served as a constant, oppressive reminder of their dehumanized status. Chattel slavery commodified their Black bodies for labor with no true regard for their basic human needs, which were compromised on many levels. There was insufficient living space, non-existent sanitation, no formal bathing facilities, or comfort in their wooden cabins. The feeling of human beings treated as property was inescapable, as described through the experience of Harriet Jacobs (1861/2001) in her seminal work *Incidents in the Life of a Slave Girl*, as she comes to understand what her family truly meant to her mistress; for the first time it sunk in that they were property, not people, as she describes here. "These God-breathing machines are no more, in the sight of their masters, than the cotton they plant, or the horses they tend."[50] This demonstrates the path of how unrelenting dehumanization can lead to chronic feelings of hopelessness, anxiety, and a diminished sense of self-worth, all compounding the physical hardships of daily life they endured.

The lack of hygiene, inadequate clothing, and overcrowded, substandard living quarters were not incidental hardships; they were deliberate mechanisms of oppression, calculated to maximize labor while minimizing investment in the well-being of enslaved people. These conditions inflicted lasting physical and psychological harm, manifesting in chronic illnesses, weakened immune systems, and premature death. The trauma of these substandard living conditions and their dehumanizing effects laid a foundation of health inequities and collective suffering that continues to reverberate in the lives of their descendants.

As a means of rising above their deplorable housing conditions, enslaved Africans demonstrated remarkable resilience by transforming these spaces into sites of cultural preservation, resistance, and familial strength. Acts of domestic life, sharing stories, practicing spiritual rituals, singing lullabies, and passing down oral histories, turned spaces of dehumanization into sacred grounds of survival and continuity. Even the physical act of maintaining cleanliness and personalizing the interior with handmade items like quilts, baskets, or religious symbols was a form of quiet defiance, asserting dignity and reclaiming a sense of ownership over their environment. In this way, the living quarters, though intentionally oppressive, became powerful symbols of resilience, where enslaved Africans sustained their identities, nurtured their communities, and laid the groundwork for future resistance.

Hunger as a Weapon

At its most basic level, nutrition is foundational to human health, supporting cellular energy, growth, and development. For enslaved Africans, however, the diet they were provided flagrantly contrasted with the nutritional needs demanded by their grueling physical labor. The rations distributed to enslaved people were not necessarily designed to sustain health or well-being; they were calculated only to maintain the bare minimum level of physical functioning required to exploit their labor. Slavery built the infrastructure of capitalism in America, where profits trump people then and now. Food, beyond housing, is one of the largest expenses today, just as it was historically. Therefore, on plantations, food was an operational expense to be minimized, often at the expense of the enslaved populations' well-being. Regardless of limited historical knowledge connecting nutrition to disease at that time, it does not change the experience the enslaved had with receiving insufficient quantity and quality of food that contributed to widespread malnutrition, compounded by their other deplorable living conditions that left them vulnerable to chronic health issues and a legacy of health disparities.

Historians Kiple & King described a typical diet of enslaved adults as consisting of weekly rations of salt pork and cornmeal, with occasional molasses, sweet potato, and fruit.[51] Although many historians differ on how much food was given to the enslaved, formerly enslaved Celestia Avery recalls her own lived experience during that time:

> *"Slaves were required to prepare their own meals three times a day. This was done in a big open fireplace which was filled with hot coals. The master did not give them much of a variety of food, but allowed each family to raise their own vegetables. Each family was given a hand out of bacon and meal on Saturdays and through the week, corn ash cakes and meat.....The diet did not vary even at Christmas only a little fruit was added."*[52]

These rations lacked the vitamins, minerals, and macronutrients necessary for proper physical health, not to mention the added nutrition needed to sustain cellular resources during their intense physical labor. Enslaved men and women were being forced to work 10-14-hour days (depending on the season) in the fields, performing labor-intensive tasks that burned thousands of calories per day. Yet, their nutritional intake was insufficient to maintain a healthy balance among heavy energetic output, leading to exhaustion, muscle wasting, and long-term health degradation. The harsh realities of this inadequate quality and quantity of their diet were vividly described by Frederick Douglass in his autobiography: "We were allowed less than a half a bushel of corn-meal per week, and very little else, either in the shape of meat or vegetables. It was not enough for us to subsist upon."[53]

Contrasted with their pre-enslavement diets in West Africa, rich in fruits, vegetables, grains, nuts, and lean proteins, the food provided during slavery was nutritionally barren. In Africa, many communities cultivated diverse diets that included millet, yams, plantains, and nuts, supplemented with medicinal herbs. Meats were typically consumed sparingly and supplemented agricultural yields, making the diet more balanced and sustainable. This nutrient-dense diet promoted vitality and supported a communal lifestyle in which food was both sustenance and a shared experience. This way of eating was not only practical but also a reflection of a deeply ingrained respect for the land and its resources, a stark contrast to the conditions they faced in America. This nutritional heritage would be lost in the transatlantic trade, replaced by a diet engineered to maximize labor efficiency at minimal cost.

"Because of their availability, low cost, and supposed nutritional value, pork and corn constituted the primary foods for Virginia slaves," according to Historian Todd Savitt.[54] This was a microcosm of dietary rations provided to the enslaved across the South that, unfortunately, left many with deficiencies in key micronutrients, including B vitamins, vitamin D, calcium, magnesium, and iron.[55] Niacin (B3) deficiency, in particular, led to pellagra, a condition characterized by the "four D's"—diarrhea, dermatitis, dementia, and death. This condition was prevalent among the enslaved who consumed corn as a staple food without other macro- and micronutrients in the diet to support daily niacin requirements. Pellagra's additional symptoms included mental confusion, weakness, and paralysis, with infected individuals reaching epidemic proportions by the mid-1840s, as evidenced by the adopted term "black tongue."[56]

Unfortunately, the nutritional deprivation extended to the more vulnerable enslaved individuals, including pregnant and nursing mothers and their children, who were also underfed. Maternal nutrition played a pivotal role in low birth weights, making enslaved infants more at risk for illness and contributing to their high infant mortality rates during the first year of life. In addition, malnourished infants and toddlers frequently suffered from stunted growth, weakened immune systems, and high mortality rates. According to the New York African Burial Ground Project, skeletal remains of enslaved children revealed conditions like rickets and porotic hyperostosis, which indicate severe malnutrition.[57] For enslaved mothers who would go on to live a labor-intensive life on the plantation and most likely endure additional pregnancies, there was no opportunity to break this cycle of malnutrition for them or their offspring. With each subsequent pregnancy, nutrition was continuing to be extracted from already nearly depleted tissue stores, creating a maternal environment of deprivation and scarcity, being a constant for both the mother and the fetus, with no opportunity to fully recover. The effects of sustained malnutrition persisted, ensuring that even those who survived passed along a legacy of nutritional inadequacy to their descendants.

The nutritional deprivation endured by enslaved Africans was not simply a matter of poor diet; it was an extension of the dehumanization they faced, another barrier that ultimately denied their bodies the necessary means to thrive. Their malnutrition was a weapon, weakening their bodies while extracting every ounce of labor possible. This deprivation was not an isolated hardship but part of a larger structure designed to deplete their humanity. Food, a fundamental human need, was wielded to assert control and maintain dependency. The inadequate amounts and diversity of nutrition dispersed amongst the enslaved reinforced the power imbalance, ensuring that enslaved individuals remained physically weakened and mentally subjugated.

Despite being inadequately nourished by enslavers, many of the enslaved demonstrated remarkable resilience by supplementing these rations through covert and strategic means. They cultivated small garden plots during their limited personal time, growing nutrient-rich foods to complement the meager rations they were given by their enslavers. They planted vegetables such as okra, sweet potatoes, and cowpeas, foods deeply tied to African culinary traditions. Others fished, foraged for wild herbs, berries, and roots, or hunted small game when circumstances allowed. These acts not only improved their nutritional intake over time but also preserved cultural foodways, passed down across generations in the face of forced displacement. Women in particular played a critical role in sustaining families by creatively preparing meals that maximized both nutrition and taste, often using communal cooking to strengthen kinship bonds. In this way, food became more than sustenance; it became a form of resistance, cultural preservation, and survival against the systemic deprivation imposed by slavery.

Conclusion

The bodies of enslaved Blacks were stripped of their humanity by social and legal systems that worked in tandem to keep them reduced to objects incapable of love, connection, intellect, creativity or spiritual depth. This system subjected their bodies to relentless brutality, which exploited their robust physical power and strength into commodified units of labor. Meanwhile, the distribution of their most basic needs of food, clothing, rest, and shelter correlated more with the maximized extraction of labor and reproduction, versus any need to support their health and well-being. This toxic environment, rooted in dehumanization and sustained by systemic neglect, gave rise to deeply harmful physical conditions that included but were not limited to: chronic exhaustion, exposure to the elements, and severe malnutrition. Over time, this produced a pattern of physical deterioration that became embedded in the Black American health narrative. And yet, the physical trauma was only the beginning. The psychological violations they endured—often invisible but just as damaging—would leave even deeper scars. These harms not only shaped the immediate suffering of the enslaved but, as we will explore in later chapters, laid the groundwork for the intergenerational transmission of disease, trauma, and health vulnerability still evident today. As science begins to catch up with what communities have long known, it is clear: the body remembers, and it carries the weight of a stolen past.

CHAPTER 3:
THE PSYCHOLOGICAL ASSAULT: TRAUMA, CONTROL, AND IDENTITY ERASURE

The institution of slavery in America relied on a systematic approach to breaking the minds, bodies, and spirits of enslaved Africans. This dehumanization was not merely a byproduct of the economic system but an intentional tool to maintain control and enforce compliance. By intertwining physical brutality with psychological trauma, enslavers constructed a framework of oppression that left no aspect of enslaved individuals' lives untouched. The simultaneous attack on the body and mind ensured that the enslaved were stripped not only of their freedom but also of their identity, autonomy, and humanity. The methods used to achieve this dehumanization were not just systematic; they were multifaceted; together, these tactics laid a psychological infrastructure that has penetrated the lives of subsequent generations in very profound and traumatic ways.

The Silencing of Culture

Central to this dehumanization was the deliberate erasure of cultural identity. Enslaved Africans were torn from their homeland, forced into a foreign environment, and subjected to a systemic process designed to sever them from their roots. This cultural erasure created a void, leaving the enslaved disconnected from their past and vulnerable to the imposed identity of inferiority (Discussed in Chapter 1) that slavery perpetuated.

Names, which held profound significance in West African culture, were systematically stripped away and replaced with those imposed by plantation owners to reflect their ownership. In West African traditions, names were not merely identifiers. However, they carried deep personal, familial, and spiritual significance, often linking individuals to their lineage, tribal affiliations, and even significant life events, such as the day of their birth. These names affirmed one's place within a community and served as a constant connection to ancestry and cultural heritage. Upon arrival in the Americas, enslaved men, women, and children were forcibly renamed, often adopting the surnames of their enslavers to signify their legal status as property. This renaming severed them from their heritage and reduced their identities to commodities. For example, a woman named Yaa Asantewaa—whose name signified her Thursday birth, identity as a warrior princess, and deep ancestral ties—might suddenly be called "Harriet," erasing any visible trace of her cultural connection. Historian Michael Gomez writes extensively in *Exchanging Our Country Marks: The Transformation of African Identities in the Colonial and Antebellum South* (1998) about how this intentional strategy disrupted the continuity of African identity and belonging amongst the enslaved.[58] This deliberate cultural disconnection served as a powerful psychological weapon, with the loss of one's name symbolizing the loss of self. Through this erasure of personal and communal identities, enslavers sought to create a blank slate upon which they could inscribe narratives of inferiority, submission, and servitude.

The loss of identity was compounded by the systematic dismantling of language. Enslaved Africans were deliberately separated from others who shared their native tongues to stifle communication, limit solidarity, and prevent the preservation of cultural practices. Without the ability to speak their languages and not knowing the English language initially, enslaved individuals were further isolated, deepening their sense of alienation and weakening their ability to resist oppression collectively.

Beyond the loss of names and language, enslaved Africans were often prohibited from practicing their traditional customs, rituals, and spiritual beliefs. These cultural practices—including storytelling, drumming, dance, and ancestor veneration—had provided vital sources of strength, healing, and communal identity. This identity conflicted with the religious and cultural beliefs of their white Christian enslavers. "Dance was to the African a means of establishing contact with the ancestors and with the gods."[59] However, such expressions were seen as sinful and often banned outright, and harsh punishments were inflicted upon those who attempted to maintain them. In addition, drums were also central to both communication and spirituality in many West African cultures and were frequently confiscated or destroyed to prevent their use in inciting acts of rebellion among the enslaved.

Religious practices faced similar suppression. The spiritual systems and rituals that had once provided enslaved Africans with guidance, protection, healing, and a deep connection to the divine were replaced with a distorted version of Christianity designed to reinforce submission. The enslaved were often told that their suffering was divinely ordained, as slaveholders manipulated biblical texts to justify bondage and obedience. This weaponized theology not only stripped away ancestral religious practices and dismantled the communal gatherings of shared cultural expressions that were central to West African societies, but it also changed the identity of who they knew God to be. Christianity became another instrument of control that enslavers used to indoctrinate listeners that slavery was biblical and a part of God's divine plan.

Cultural erasure was not incidental but a strategic method of domination, designed to sever enslaved Africans from their past while limiting their ability to imagine futures beyond enslavement. The relentless psychological assault of having their identities dismantled led many to internalize feelings of worthlessness, inferiority, and despair. Without access to the cultural frameworks that once affirmed their humanity, many enslaved individuals experienced profound disorientation and hopelessness. Denying the enslaved population the ability to culturally express themselves was an attempt to sever their connections to any external tools of self-empowerment and identity.

Fortunately for the enslaved, a spiritual connection to the divine can never be severed. Even amid calculated erasure, enslaved Africans demonstrated profound resilience by preserving, adapting, and reinventing their cultural practices under the harshest of conditions. Though torn from their homelands and scattered across plantations with others of different ethnic and linguistic backgrounds, they retained elements of African traditions through music, dance, language patterns, spirituality, cuisine, and naming practices. Spirituals and ring shouts, for example, preserved African rhythms and communal worship styles while adapting to the constraints of forced Christianity, becoming both expressions of faith and cultural continuity. Enslaved people created new creole languages and dialects that blended African linguistic structures with English, allowing for both communication and cultural preservation. In their food, they preserved ancestral ingredients and cooking methods, giving rise to culinary traditions that still endure today. Through hair styling, folk medicine, storytelling, and the preservation of oral histories, the enslaved affirmed their roots and passed on their cultural identity to the best of their ability to new generations. These acts were not just survival mechanisms; they were deliberate, creative expressions of resistance that kept African heritage alive in the face of brutal efforts to erase it.

Stripped of Autonomy

From the moment of their capture, enslaved Africans lost all agency over their lives, falling victim to a systematic denial of personal autonomy. They were bought and sold like livestock, stripped of the right to make even the most basic decisions about their bodies, their labor, their futures, and the futures of their descendants.

This denial of autonomy functioned as both a physical and psychological assault designed to reinforce their status as property rather than human beings. The auction block was a stark and public stage of this dehumanization, where enslaved men, women, and children were forced to stand naked or barely clothed under the scrutinizing gazes of potential buyers. Their bodies were poked, prodded, and examined as if they were merchandise, with no regard for their dignity or humanity. Historian Walter Johnson (1999) highlights how these appraisals "alienated slaves from their own bodies" as they were priced according to age, strength, and reproduction/breeding potential for those working in the fields and civility for those serving in the house.[60] The auction block was not only a site of physical violation but also a location of immense psychological trauma as they were forced to participate in their own commodification.

This complete control extended into every facet of enslaved life. The enslaved were dictated when to wake, eat, sleep, and work. They had no say over how their labor was used or the conditions under which they worked. Every hour of their day, from "can't see to can't see" (sunup to sundown), was controlled by enslavers, with severe punishments for any perceived disobedience or underperformance. The threat and reality of brutal punishments—whippings, mutilations, and executions—ensured submission and reinforced that enslaved bodies existed solely for the purposes of the enslavers' benefits, not their own. Frederick Douglass poignantly described the relentlessness of forced labor, writing, "We worked in all weathers, it was never too hot, too cold; it could never rain, blow, hail, or snow, too hard for us to work in the field. Work, work, work. The longest days were too short for him [the enslaver], and the shortest nights too long for him."[61] This relentless exploitation ensured that enslaved Africans were physically exhausted and mentally oppressed, leaving little space or strength for resistance.

Enslaved individuals lived under constant surveillance, with every aspect of their existence dictated by enslavers. The inability to make even the smallest decisions for themselves steadily eroded their

PART I: HISTORICAL FOUNDATIONS OF DEHUMANIZATION

sense of self, agency, and identity. This systematic disempowerment was not incidental—it was strategic. Enslavers deliberately intertwined physical violence with psychological control to maintain dominance and suppress resistance. By instilling feelings of helplessness and dependency, enslavers fostered internalized oppression, making the act of resistance seem impossible and survival contingent upon submission. Enslavers used the denial of autonomy as a system to ensure optimal compliance, resulting in not only economic control but also a psychological barrier for the enslaved. Such a deliberate strategy sustained the institution of slavery by breaking both the bodies and spirits of those it enslaved. It instilled in them a sense of powerlessness and dependency, eroding the individual's sense of self and making resistance seem futile. The psychological scars of being denied the right to control their own bodies or destinies were immeasurable, thereby reshaping one's definition of what freedom meant for them, as captured by former enslaved Ezra Adams, where survival superseded a need for freedom.

> *"You ain't gwine to believe dat de slaves on our plantation didn't stop workin' for old marster, even when they was told dat they was free. Us didn't want no more freedom than us was gittin' on our plantation already. Us knowed too well dat us was well took care of, wid a plenty of vittles to eat and tight log and board houses to live in. De slaves, where I lived, knowed after de war dat they had abundance of dat somethin' called freedom, what they could not eat, wear, and sleep in. Yes, sir, they soon found out dat freedom ain't nothin', 'less you is got somethin' to live on and a place to call home. Dis livin' on liberty is lak young folks livin' on love after they gits married. It just don't work. No, sir, its las' so long and not a bit longer. Don't tell me! It sho' don't hold good when you has to work, or when you gets hungry. You know dat poor white folks and niggers has got to work to live, regardless of liberty, love, and all them things. I believes a person loves more better, when they feels good. I knows from experience dat poor folks feels better when they has food in deir frame and a*

few dimes to jingle in deir pockets. I know what it means to be a nigger, wid nothin'."[62]

Despite being stripped of nearly all legal and personal autonomy, the enslaved found ways to defy plantation boundaries and white control. They practiced covert resistance to regain control over their time and bodies, including feigning illness, slowing work, or manipulating the expectations of enslavers to negotiate slightly better conditions. Additionally, they carved out spiritual spaces through secret religious gatherings known as "invisible institutions," where they preached liberation and hope, independent of the slaveholder's version of Christianity.[63] Such everyday acts of resistance as these became a way of life, a means to silently declare autonomy and resilience while affirming their personhood in a society built to intentionally tear them down.

Fractured Kinship

"Are the dearest friends and relations, now rendered more dear by their separation from their kindred, still to be parted from each other, and thus prevented from cheering the gloom of slavery, with the small comfort of being together, and mingling their sufferings and sorrows? Why are parents to lose their children, brothers their sisters, or husbands their wives? Surely, this is a new refinement in cruelty, which, while it has no advantage to atone for it, thus aggravates distress, and adds fresh horrors even to the wretchedness of slavery."[64]

The systematic destruction of families was one of the most devastating tools of dehumanization inflicted upon the enslaved. Family represents the foundation of human connection, identity, and emotional support, offering guidance, love, and a sense of belonging that are vital to self-worth and empowerment. Enslavers, fully aware of the strength that family ties provided, deliberately targeted these bonds to weaken enslaved communities and ensure submission. By dismantling the family unit, they severed the most basic sources of emotional resilience, leaving individuals isolated and vulnerable.

PART I: HISTORICAL FOUNDATIONS OF DEHUMANIZATION

For enslaved parents, the constant threat of separation from their children was a source of unrelenting anguish. At any moment, children could be sold, often without warning or the chance for a final goodbye. This agony would cut deeper than death, when children were forcefully removed from their parents, the loss was not accompanied by the potential solace of a funeral or gravesite to visit; instead, only "the searing, lasting memory of confusion and pain."[65] These separations were not incidental outcomes of the slave economy but intentional acts of cruelty designed to break emotional bonds and prevent collective resistance. Historian Heather Williams (2012) writes, "Not everyone was strong and resilient....some people broke under the pain of separation, became depressed, considered suicide, or lost their minds because they could not clear their heads of the cries of their lost children."[66] Enslavers were able to benefit from their strength being reduced to despair and brokenheartedness as a sign of surrender and yielding to control.

Unfortunately, children ripped from their parents were thrust into environments devoid of comfort, guidance, and unconditional love. Psychologists have long understood the devastating effects of such early trauma. Psychologist John Bowlby, in his research on attachment theory, emphasizes the connection between prolonged separation from the primary caregiver in early childhood and how it can result in emotional detachment, anxiety, and difficulty forming secure relationships later in life.[67] Similarly, van der Kolk writes, "Children who lack stable attachments develop survival strategies rooted in fear, mistrust, and emotional numbness, impairing their ability to thrive."[68] These insights help affirm what enslaved people endured: that the psychological wounds from family separations left scars that shaped not only childhood but an individual's entire life—leaving the minds of enslaved children to become even more suggestive to the conditioning of their enslavers when their parents were not around to provide a counter-narrative or understanding of life.

Beyond physical separations, enslaved parents were stripped of the ability to nurture and guide their children. Enslavers denied them the chance to pass on cultural traditions, familial wisdom, and communal values. As a result, many enslaved children grew up severed not only from their parents but from their cultural heritage. Parenting was a point of exposure to connection, identity, and culture that many children lacked. As a result, these disruptions fostered deep psychological wounds rooted in rejection, abandonment, and loss. Torn from the only sources of safety and love they knew, these children were left to navigate hostile environments alone. Their identities were shaped by trauma rather than tradition and disconnection rather than belonging. Esteemed author bell hooks reflects on how being denied the right to belong equates to being denied the right to be fully human due to the severity of its impact on personal well-being.[69] This undoubtedly further fostered an environment of dehumanization.

The destruction extended beyond the selling of children away from their parents and vice versa. By separating spouses, siblings, and extended family, enslavers dismantled entire community support systems. The resulting fragmentation weakened the collective strength of enslaved people, ensuring their focus remained on survival rather than rebellion. Witnessing the repeated loss of others' loved ones created an atmosphere of constant fear and despair, reinforcing feelings of powerlessness and hopelessness. Such a deliberate dismantling of enslaved families left a lasting legacy of trauma that reverberates through generations. The loss of familial bonds, cultural knowledge, and belonging disrupted the natural development of identity and community. Today, these historical wounds persist in stereotypes rooted in slavery, such as the absent Black father or the hyper-independent Black mother. These harmful narratives ignore the historical realities of forced family separations and instead pathologize the very survival strategies born from such conditions.

Regardless of persistent violent disruptions to their family, the enslaved demonstrated extraordinary resilience by continuously reconstructing and preserving family bonds in both blood and chosen forms. Enslaved parents instilled cultural values, spiritual beliefs, and survival skills in their children, often under threat of punishment, ensuring the transmission of identity and heritage. When biological families were torn apart, enslaved individuals created extended kin networks and fictive kin relationships, referring to one another as "brother," "sister," "auntie," "uncle," or "cousin," rebuilding systems of care and emotional support.[70] These relationships functioned as protective structures, offering guidance, discipline, and affection in environments designed to erode human connection. Moreover, with love being the strongest force in the universe, many undertook extraordinary risks to reunite with family members, traveling long distances, negotiating with enslavers, or escaping slavery altogether to find lost loved ones. These efforts to maintain and restore familial bonds were not only acts of love but also powerful assertions of humanity, identity, and resistance in a world intent on erasing them.

Gendered Brutality

The emasculation of enslaved men was a deliberate and multifaceted strategy designed not only to dominate and control but also to dismantle the social and psychological fabric of enslaved communities. Through relentless physical violence, sexual exploitation, and psychological warfare, enslavers systematically stripped men of their traditional roles as protectors, providers, and leaders. This targeted dehumanization reduced them to tools of labor and reproduction, erasing their autonomy, dignity, and identity.

The bodies of enslaved men became ongoing sites of terror, where violence was enacted not only as punishment but as a form of psychological control. Enslaved men endured brutal beatings with whips, chains, and other weapons, leaving lasting scars that served both as personal reminders of their subjugation and public warnings to deter resistance. Shackles and irons physically restrained their movements, while branding irons seared flesh with the marks of ownership, reducing human beings to living property. Lynchings became a particularly brutal spectacle, used not only to punish but to publicly humiliate and terrorize enslaved populations. Formerly enslaved, J.F. Boone painfully describes these horrific acts as he recalls, "The overseer was pretty cruel. My father has seen them whipped till they couldn't stand up and then salt and things that hurt poured into their wounds."[71] In most cases, the stronger the will of the man, the more brutal and deliberate the violence against him.

The magnitude of savage beatings would vary, sometimes with the violence ceasing at the doorsteps of death and sometimes crossing the actual threshold. Regardless of severity, the purpose was usually the same, meant to be painful, shameful, and exemplary to other slaves, a reminder of who held the true power. These acts were often carried out in full view of other enslaved individuals, including family members and children, ensuring the psychological trauma extended well beyond the individual victim. Formerly enslaved Rev. W.B. Allen recounts the various reasons the enslaved would be prematurely forced to go meet their maker. He states that, "I have personally known a few slaves that were beaten to death for one or more of the follow offenses: leaving home without a pass, talking back to - 'sassing' - a white person, hitting another Negro, fussing, fighting, and rukkussing in the quarters, lying, loitering on their work, taking things - the whites called it stealing."[72] Lastly, former enslaved, Andy Anderson, discusses how the abuse made him feel after being punished for mistakenly rolling a wheelbarrow into a tree stump and breaking it. He recalls, "He ties me to the stake and every half hour for four hours, dey lays ta lashes on my back. For de first couple hours de pain am awful. I's never forgot it. Den I's stood so much pain I not feel so much and when dey taks me loose, I's us' 'bout half dead. I lays in de bund two days, gittin' over dat whippin', gittin' over it in de body but not de heart. No, suh, I has dat in de heart till dis day."[73] Andy's physical wounds may have healed but it left behind a trail of emotional scars.

Nonetheless, among the most extreme forms of violence not resulting in physical death was castration, designed to destroy not

PART I: HISTORICAL FOUNDATIONS OF DEHUMANIZATION

only the physical autonomy of enslaved men but their perceived masculinity and reproductive power. Often overlooked in historical narratives is that enslaved men were also victims of sexual violence. Through forced breeding, men were compelled to impregnate multiple women purely for the economic benefit of their enslavers. "Men recalled being treated like breeding animals. Men were selected specifically for raising up strong black bucks."[74] These forced pairings stripped enslaved men of the ability to form genuine relationships and rendered them biological instruments rather than human beings with desires, attachments, and agency. In addition, although much attention has rightly been given to the sexual exploitation of enslaved women, enslaved men were also subjected to rape and sexual assault by the hands of their by male and female enslavers. This rarely discussed form of control is highlighted throughout the documentary "Buck Breaking" as it reviews how breaking enslaved men sexually and through other forms of violence was used to completely strip them of their manhood, autonomy, and their ability to resist, reinforcing the total power of the enslaver over their lives.[75]

Motivated by domination and complete control, enslavers used other harrowing tactics to psychologically break enslaved men by forcing them to witness the abuse of their loved ones. Men were routinely made to watch the sexual assault or brutal beating of their wives, daughters, or sisters, entirely powerless to intervene. As explained by white, "Black women, unfortunately, proved to be mirrors for black men. Each time the former was abused, the latter's own helplessness was reflected."[76] This orchestrated helplessness not only inflicted deep psychological trauma among the enslaved men but also further eroded their sense of masculinity and self-worth. They were treated as if they were void of human value, worth, or emotions. In many cases, they were only sperm donors with no legal or social power to protect even the children they could acknowledge. Enslaved men were not heartless; they felt the ever-present threat of family separation that loomed over their lives, as children and partners could be sold away at any given moment. This systemic destabilization dismantled any semblance of their paternal authority or protection, leaving them feeling powerless and stripped of their fundamental roles as fathers and husbands.

The physical and psychological trauma inflicted upon enslaved men was deeply intertwined. Acts of physical violence—whippings, brandings, castrations, and lynching—were intentionally public, serving as both punishment and spectacle. These events instilled fear and submission while simultaneously reinforcing feelings of inadequacy and helplessness. This systematic dehumanization worked to isolate enslaved men not only from their families and communities but from their own identities. Over time, constant exposure to degradation and inferiority narratives created internal conflicts, as enslaved men struggled to reconcile their innate sense of worth with the societal message and demonstration of their subjugation. Frantz Fanon depicts in *Black Skin, White Masks (2008),* how the colonized man internalizes his own inferiority and his psyche becomes molded by the gaze of the oppressor.[77] All of which makes it difficult to excel beyond such limitations without intentional introductions to a new narrative. Unfortunately, these psychological wounds did not end with emancipation. The legacy of emasculation persisted, shaping post-slavery dynamics around Black masculinity, fatherhood, and leadership. The trauma embedded in generations of forced subjugation, violence, and public humiliation has continued to influence the roles and identities of Black men in families and society.

Although they faced relentless assaults on their humanity, enslaved men exhibited profound resilience. As recognized by Ralph Ellison as he speaks of the resilience of the enslaved, "Any people who could endure all of that brutalization and keep together, who could undergo such dismemberment and resuscitate itself and endure until it could take the initiative in achieving its own freedom is obviously more than the sum of its brutalization."[78] Many bodies may have been broken, but not their collective spirits. They resisted through overt and covert acts of defiance, maintaining family bonds where possible, and quietly asserted their humanity in the midst of systemic degradation. The survival of enslaved men and the preservation of cultural, familial, and communal identity stand as testaments to their enduring strength and resistance. Their ability to retain dignity amid a system designed to strip it away speaks to the unbreakable aspects of the human spirit, even under the most brutal conditions.

Sexual Violence of Enslaved Women

Echoing the treatment of men, enslaved women were also handled like commodities, only to be used as tools for labor, reproduction, and sexual exploitation. The targeted control and violation of their bodies served both economic and ideological purposes, fueling the growth of slavery while reinforcing white supremacy and the systemic devaluation of Black womanhood. Every fraction of their physical bodies was used for the complete satisfaction and advancement of the enslavers, leaving the enslaved women disconnected from their own sense of womanhood and self-worth.

Treating a woman as if her body does not belong to her and therefore, that which comes from her body does not belong to her either, is an act of physical, sexual, and psychological violence. Enslaved women were systematically stripped of their roles as mothers and caregivers, reduced instead to instruments of reproduction to sustain and expand the enslaved population, particularly after the abolition of the Transatlantic Slave Trade in 1808. Under this system, women were forced into pregnancies year after year, often paired with men without consent, and subjected to unrelenting physical labor even while pregnant. Their existence carried a double burden of laborer and reproducer as explained by historian Deborah Gray White, "Female slavery had much to do with work, but much of it was concerned with bearing, nourishing, and rearing children whom slaveholders needed for the continual replenishment of their labor force."[79] The toll of this duality in roles was unrelenting to their mind, body, and spirit.

This cruelty extended to their children, who were frequently sold away, particularly once they reached working age severing maternal bonds and leaving permanent psychological scars.[80] To further deepen the emotional injury, enslaved women were often forced to serve as wet nurses for the children of their enslavers. This exploitation required them to provide nourishment to white infants while their own children were neglected or sold off to other plantations. The emotional toll of feeding the children of those who enslaved and brutalized them, while being denied the right to care for their own, created a deep sense of grief and helplessness. This practice reinforced the total control enslavers exerted over every aspect of their bodies, from reproduction to sustenance.

The physical and psychological trauma of forced reproduction was inexorable, especially when compounded with the physical exhaustion of the fields and malnutrition, all of which led to high rates of miscarriage and maternal mortality. Personal accounts further illuminate these atrocities, as formerly enslaved Mary Ann John recalls one of her mother's birthing experiences on the plantation: "You see, what caused my ma to be sickly, I was de oldest child, and dey made her work too hard with de other children. One of my sisters was born right in de fields. Dey just dug two holes, one in the front and one in the back. She gets down in dat hole and give birth to de baby; de baby just rolls out in de hole. Den de boss has someone to take the baby to the house, and makes my ma get up and keep right on hoeing. I never will forget."[81] Although maternity leave was not a concept at the time for a minimum of six weeks off, Mary Ann's mother was not given six hours of recovery before resuming work obligations. This further exemplifies how enslaved women were not humans giving birth to infants but were treated as if they were machines producing more bodies to be commodified for the benefit of the enslavers.

Sexual violence was a pervasive and deliberate tool of control inflicted upon enslaved women that was not only limited to breeding practices, which historian Diana Ramey Berry refers to as "third-par-

PART I: HISTORICAL FOUNDATIONS OF DEHUMANIZATION

ty rape."[82] Nonetheless, they were also subjected to sexual abuse by enslavers, overseers, and other white men in power. Therefore, rape was a common occurrence within institutionalized slavery, used as a way to assert dominance and economic exploitation against enslaved women. The children born from these assaults, often labeled as "mulatto," represented the physical evidence of systemic sexual violence. These children were rarely acknowledged by their white fathers and, by law, inherited the status of enslavement through their mothers, ensuring the system's perpetuation. Colorism also emerged from these dynamics, as lighter-skinned enslaved individuals were sometimes given marginally better treatment, fostering division within the enslaved community.

For enslaved women, the psychological toll of sexual violence was profound. Living under constant threat of assault and then having it compounded with the other elements of enslavement forced many to develop complex coping mechanisms to endure day after day, year after year, lifetime after lifetime. white poses the question, "Given what we know today about the effects of abuse, the way it spans feelings of anger, low self-esteem, depression, and even self-hatred, can we discuss black female survival without tackling the rage that dwelled within?"[83] Consistent with denying the humanity of Black women, their historical pain and contemporary ramifications are not only ignored but stigmatized, therefore intensifying systemic barriers that hinder access to support and healing resources. Just as the present is a reflection of the past, as a means of survival, Black women are left to normalize their internal and external scars with little to no reprieve, at the expense of their health.

The hyper-sexualization and abuse of enslaved women's bodies were not isolated acts of cruelty; they were embedded into the very structure of slavery. Despite being denied the right to consent, to protect their children, and to control their own bodies, enslaved women resisted erasure of their identities. They knew that they were more than commodities to be bought and sold on the slave market. They found ways to navigate the unrelenting assault on their dignity and displayed remarkable acts of strength and resilience. Through acts of quiet defiance, solidarity with other women, and the preservation of cultural practices and stories, they fought through blood, sweat, and tears to maintain their humanity. Their survival and the survival of their descendants stand as profound testaments to the strength and endurance of the human spirit under unimaginable oppression.

The height of a determined woman's resilience is recounted by formerly enslaved Celestia Avery as she tells of her enslaved grandmother surviving the viciousness of her slave master, who brutally whipped her for praying. A practice he deeply despised because slaves prayed in hopes of freedom for themselves, which seemed to trigger his deepest fear.

> *The master heard her and became so angry he came to her cabin, seized and pulled her clothes from her body and tied her to a young sapling. He whipped her so brutally that her body was raw all over. When darkness fell her husband cut her down from the tree, during the day he was afraid to go near her. Rather than go back to the cabin she crawled on her knees to the woods and her husband brought grease for her raw body. For two weeks the master hunted but could not find her; however, when he finally did, she had given birth to twins. The only thing that saved her was the fact that she was a mid-wife and always carried a small pin knife which she used to cut the navel cord of the babies. After doing this she tore her petticoat into two pieces and wrapped each baby. Grandmother Sylvia lived to get 115 years old.*[84]

The lived experience of Celestia's grandmother did not allow her time to grieve and feel sorry for her abuse; the duty of motherhood called her name, and she answered "yes" every day for a long life far beyond the average life expectancy.

PART I: HISTORICAL FOUNDATIONS OF DEHUMANIZATION

Weaponization of Stereotypes

Central to the dehumanization of the enslaved was the deliberate creation and perpetuation of negative labels and stereotypes. These damaging narratives were essential in justifying the system of slavery and reinforcing the social hierarchy that positioned Africans and their descendants as inherently inferior. Stereotypes functioned not only as external tools of control but also as internal mechanisms of psychological oppression, limiting how the enslaved were perceived by society at large and, over time, influencing how they began to perceive themselves and others who looked like them.

Throughout slavery, enslaved Africans were systematically labeled as subhuman, lazy, uncivilized, and hypersexual—dangerous caricatures designed to rationalize exploitation and violence. These stereotypes were projected onto their physical features—dark skin, broad noses, full hips, lips, and buttocks—which were disparaged as unfavorable traits of beauty and used as visual markers of supposed biological inferiority, backed by pseudoscientific theories (discussed in Chapter 1). The darker the skin, the more one was associated with savagery and primitiveness, reinforcing a racial hierarchy that placed whiteness as the ideal and Blackness as a deformity of the human standard.[85] Facial features, hair texture, and body type were also scrutinized and caricatured in popular media, religious doctrine, and scientific literature to strip the enslaved of individuality and reduce them to demeaning, monolithic representations. These constructed images served to justify their mistreatment and solidify white supremacy as a social and biological order.

A long-standing, very destructive stereotype was that of hypersexuality, particularly imposed on Black women. This narrative portrayed enslaved women as naturally promiscuous and sexually insatiable, thereby justifying the rampant sexual violence they suffered at the hands of white men. Harriet Jacobs captures the horrific gendered dimension of enslavement, writing, "Slavery is terrible for men, but it is far more terrible for women. Superadded to the burden common to all, they have wrongs, and sufferings, and mortifications peculiarly their own... If God has bestowed beauty upon her, it will prove her greatest curse. That which commands admiration in the white women only hastens the degradation of the female slave."[86] This stereotype absolved enslavers of responsibility by blaming women with no autonomy for their assaults, which reinforced the perception that Black women were somehow unworthy of innocence, chastity, or protection.

Black men were commonly stereotyped as inherently violent, aggressive, and hypermasculine, traits used to justify extreme surveillance and brutal punishment. Yet in a cruel contradiction, enslavers often provoked and punished the very qualities they feared: leadership, intelligence, and resistance. As historian, Walter Johnson explains, "These slaves were bought to be broken, to be turned from unruly subjects into perfect symbols of their owners' will. Indeed, they were bought to be the embodied registers of the indomitability of that will, for the slaves themselves were the ultimate audience for their buyers' brutal performances."[87] Strength and autonomy—normally admired traits—were twisted into signs of danger when displayed by Black men, reinforcing a dehumanizing logic that cast their potential for empowerment as a threat. This dichotomy not only justified violence but also upheld the false narrative that Black masculinity was inherently dangerous and in need of constant control.

The stigmatization of African physical features was not only used to enforce a racial hierarchy between whites and Blacks but also to divide the enslaved population itself. Enslavers often favored lighter-skinned individuals—those with features closer to European standards—over those with darker skin, assigning them relatively less grueling labor assignments, such as work in the household rather than the fields. This division laid the foundation for colorism, a form of discrimination based on skin tone within the Black community. Scholar Evelyn Nakano Glenn recognizes how colorism operated as a divisive strategy, producing internal stratification and weakening group cohesion among the enslaved.[88] By privileging proximity to whiteness, enslavers deepened social fractures that would persist long after emancipation. Although some lighter-skinned enslaved individuals may have experienced marginally better conditions, colorism ultimately served the interests of the oppressors by fostering jealousy, distrust, and disunity. The legacy of this intra-group stratification remains deeply entrenched in African American communities today, with measurable effects on social and economic outcomes.

The stereotypes and labels born during slavery did not end with emancipation. Instead, they evolved, shaping modern systems of anti-Black racism that continue to harm African Americans in every facet of life. Contemporary media often reproduces these harmful archetypes, portraying Black women as hypersexual or domineering and Black men as dangerous or criminal. These portrayals have real-world consequences, from employment discrimination to racial profiling and disproportionate policing. In addition, studies have shown that negative stereotypes continue to influence perceptions and behaviors, also leading to disparities in healthcare, education, and the criminal justice system.[89] What is truly detrimental to the Black community is that the internalization of these stereotypes contributes to what psychologist Frantz Fanon identified as "epidermalization"–the process by which the oppressed come to embody the negative perceptions imposed upon them, often leading to chronic feelings of inadequacy, self-doubt, and hopelessness.[90] The psychological toll of centuries of being labeled inferior, with every aspect of societal infrastructure reinforcing the concept, is immeasurable. These stereotypes were definitely more than just words; they were tools of oppression that continue to shape identities, behaviors, and life outcomes (this topic is discussed further in the Social Identity Barrier of Part II).

In response to the deeply entrenched negative labels and stereotypes that portrayed them as intellectually inferior, morally deficient, or naturally suited for servitude, the enslaved demonstrated powerful forms of resilience by cultivating counter-narratives through culture, intellect, and spirituality. Though denied formal education, many risked punishment to secretly learn to read and write, recognizing literacy as a pathway to empowerment and resistance. Enslaved artisans, musicians, midwives, and holistic natural healers preserved and elevated African knowledge systems, skills, and traditions, showcasing their intellectual complexity and cultural richness despite being verbally branded as uncivilized or primitive. Spirituality also served as a refuge and a form of resistance; through the reinterpretation of Christian messages of liberation, enslaved people reclaimed a sense of self-worth and divine purpose that defied the dehumanizing ideologies imposed upon them. Through storytelling, naming practices, and the oral transmission of ancestral wisdom, they affirmed their identity and humanity, dismantling the legitimacy of racist stereotypes from within the confines of bondage. These acts were not only forms of survival but also radical assertions of dignity and self-definition in the face of constant psychological assault.

Denied Knowledge

One of the most insidious tools of dehumanization used by enslavers was the systematic denial of education to the enslaved. Education is a pathway to self-empowerment, critical thinking, and resistance to oppression. Enslavers understood this, which is why they enacted laws and brutal practices to keep enslaved people in a state of enforced ignorance, ensuring dependency, submission, and the perpetuation of white supremacy. As the late Toni Morrison reminds us, "if you can only be tall because somebody is on their knees, then you have a serious problem." The deliberate suppression of education not only controlled the enslaved population but also helped sustain the myth of Black intellectual inferiority as a basis for white supremacy, a narrative designed to justify the economic and social structures of slavery.

Throughout the antebellum South, literacy among enslaved people was not merely discouraged—it was criminalized. State slave codes codified these restrictions, imposing severe penalties on anyone who dared to educate enslaved individuals. For example, South

Carolina's 1740 Slave Code warned that "the education of slaves tends to excite dissatisfaction in their minds and produce insurrection and rebellion."[91] This language directly linked literacy to the potential for resistance, reinforcing the enslavers' fears that knowledge would disrupt the system that relied on subjugation.

These legal barriers were enforced through violence and terror. Enslaved people caught reading, writing, or attempting to teach others faced brutal punishments, including whippings, mutilation, imprisonment, and death. One North Carolina newspaper posted, "According to the law of North Carolina enacted in 1831, to teach a slave to read or write, or sell or give him any book or pamphlet is punished with thirty nine lashes or imprisonment, if the offender be free negro; but if a white, then with a fine of $200 (approximately $6500 today)."[92] Louisiana's penalty was even steeper, as written in the Green Mountain Freeman: "In Louisiana, the penalty of instructing a free black in a Sunday School is for the first offense, $500 (equivalent of $16,000 today); for the second, death!"[93] The very act of reading—a fundamental human right—became a radical and subversive act under slavery. Enslavers understood that a literate enslaved population threatened their control, as literacy was not just about communication but about consciousness and the ability to envision freedom. As recorded by Frederick Douglass, "Indeed, he advised me to complete thoughtlessness of the future and taught me to depend solely upon him for happiness. He seemed to see fully the pressing necessity of setting aside my intellectual nature, in order to contentment in slavery. But in spite of him, and even in spite of myself, I continued to think and to think about the injustice of my enslavement and the means of escape."[94]

The denial of education was more than a practical tool of oppression; it was a psychological weapon designed to strip enslaved people of agency and hope. By systematically blocking access to knowledge, enslavers reinforced the narrative that African-descended people were intellectually inferior and inherently incapable of self-governance. This created a deeply embedded cycle of dependency in which enslaved individuals were forced to rely on their oppressors for information, instruction, and survival.

The psychological toll of this deprivation was profound. To be denied the right to learn was to be denied the ability to imagine a future beyond enslavement. Paulo Freire explains in *Pedagogy of the Oppressed* that dehumanization can establish itself as oppression through the denial of the right to speak one's word, to express one's consciousness, and thereby to become fully human.[95] For the enslaved, literacy represented more than letters on a page; it was the key to reclaiming selfhood and possibility. Adding to the cruelty, enslavers projected the consequences of this enforced ignorance back onto the enslaved, framing their lack of education as evidence of natural inferiority. This narrative justified not only their continued enslavement but also later societal exclusions from political participation, economic opportunity, and intellectual life—stereotypes that persist today.

The denial of education did not end with emancipation. After slavery, African Americans continued to face systemic barriers to learning, from Black Codes restricting their freedom to segregated and underfunded schools under Jim Crow. These structural inequalities reinforced the legacy of slavery, creating educational disparities that persist today. Furthermore, the myth of intellectual inferiority, rooted in the deliberate denial of education, continues to shape societal attitudes about African American academic achievement and potential. Despite centuries of evidence of high intelligence, intellectual deficiency continues to be used as a durable justification for inequitable academic resources and access, according to Jarvis Givens in his book *Fugitive Pedagogy (2021)*.[96] Noteworthy contributions in science, literature, technology, medicine, arts, and entertainment continue to be viewed as the exception and not the standard for African Americans excelling despite inequitable academic conditions.

Stretching beyond the barriers in front of them that could even lead to death, the enslaved displayed extraordinary resilience by

PART I: HISTORICAL FOUNDATIONS OF DEHUMANIZATION

seeking knowledge in secret gatherings, known as "pit schools"—organized in the woods, cabins, and other hidden spaces where literacy was shared in whispers and candlelight.[97] As a quiet act of self-empowerment, they learned to read and write at great personal risk because they understood the value of knowledge. Many were taught by sympathetic whites, other enslaved individuals, or self-taught through observation and creativity, using Bible pages, scraps of newspapers, or letters as learning tools. Literacy became both a symbol and a tool of resistance, allowing them to forge passes, read abolitionist literature, communicate covertly, and eventually participate in movements for liberation and justice. Enslaved people also passed on oral traditions, stories, and proverbs, using them as educational tools to transmit values, history, and cultural knowledge when formal instruction was inaccessible. Even when denied books, they turned to memory, music, and storytelling to create intellectual legacies. These defiant acts of learning were powerful assertions of self-worth and vision, laying the groundwork for future generations to continue the pursuit of freedom and equality through education that continued after the Proclamation of Emancipation. From the establishment of Historically Black Colleges and Universities (HBCUs) during Reconstruction to the student-led protests of the Civil Rights Movement, African Americans continually utilized education as a tool of liberation and empowerment.

Conclusion

The physical and psychological trauma of dehumanization inflicted upon enslaved Africans was profound despite its being normalized by society and sanctioned by law. What we now label as abuse, exploitation, neglect, and violence—acts that rightly provoke collective outrage today—were daily realities for those forced into bondage. Stripped of their humanity, enslaved Africans endured systemic violence that not only wounded the body but fractured the mind and spirit. As scholars like James and Anderson have shown, the forced separation of families, the denial of bodily autonomy, and the relentless reinforcement of inferiority through physical punishment and psychological manipulation created a legacy of intergenerational trauma.[98] This trauma, though rarely acknowledged in its historical context, left deep scars that did not disappear with emancipation—they were encoded in memory, behavior, and even the body itself.

Central to this trauma was the deliberate construction of a false narrative of biological inferiority—an ideology that functioned as both the justification for slavery and the social glue that kept it intact. Enslavers and pro-slavery intellectuals used pseudoscience, such as craniometry and phrenology, to argue that African people were mentally and morally inferior by nature. These distorted beliefs, promoted through education, religion, law, and medicine, created a social environment where Black inferiority and white superiority were seen not just as cultural constructs but as immutable truths. This dehumanizing ideology made the enslavement of bodies of African origin appear natural and necessary. The narrative became that they were inherently "fit for servitude" and therefore unworthy of basic human rights or empathy. By embedding these lies into the very fabric of society, the institution of slavery ensured that its violence and injustice would not only be accepted but vigorously defended. This further entrenched people of African descent in a caste of perpetual subjugation and social degradation. The psychological toll of being reduced to a subhuman category was compounded by the daily reality of living in a world built to reflect and reinforce that lie.

Contemporary science affirms what enslaved Africans cellularly experienced: trauma lives in the body. As van der Kolk notes, the body quite literally "keeps the score," storing the physiological effects of fear, violence, and degradation long after the events have passed.[99] Chronic exposure to trauma has been linked to inflammation, disrupted immune function, and altered stress hormone regulation—biological responses still seen at disproportionate rates in African American communities today.[100] The epigenetic impact of slavery, compounded by generations of racial oppression, reveals that dehumanization was not just a social or moral injury—it was a

PART I: HISTORICAL FOUNDATIONS OF DEHUMANIZATION

physical one (Discussed in Part III). The body also keeps an equally powerful record of survival, resistance, and resilience. To acknowledge trauma is not to define African Americans through suffering but to affirm the strength it has taken to endure, resist, and keep on keeping on throughout the centuries.

For guided discussion questions and activities, visit: ***https://wellnessedu.blackcellconsulting.com*** *to access your FREE REFLECTION GUIDE.*

PART II
STRUCTURAL BARRIERS TO WELLNESS

PART II STRUCTURAL BARRIERS TO WELLNESS

Health is more than the absence of disease; it is the result of a complex interplay between biology, behavior, and the social environments in which individuals live, work, and play. The World Health Organization defines social determinants of health as the conditions in which people are born, grow, live, work, and age, and these determinants account for a significant portion of health disparities. For African Americans, these determinants are deeply influenced by systemic racism, embedded in every facet of society, from housing and education to access to healthcare and economic opportunity. Anti-Black racism has shaped the infrastructure of the United States, creating structural inequities that systematically disadvantage minority populations, more specifically Black communities. These inequities not only limit access to resources but also perpetuate health disparities that span generations. This part will explore how social determinants of health intersect with anti-Black racism to create environments that undermine the physical, mental, and social well-being of African Americans' ability to thrive in life fully.

BARRIER ONE:
HOUSING AND THE GEOGRAPHY OF INJUSTICE

Housing is a fundamental determinant of health, influencing physical, mental, and emotional well-being. The ability to access safe, affordable, and stable housing affects economic security, community building, and overall life expectancy. However, for African Americans, the legacy of racialized housing policies and ongoing discriminatory practices has significantly restricted homeownership, neighborhood investment, and generational wealth accumulation. These systemic housing barriers continue to shape health outcomes in the Black community, creating disparities in disease prevalence, stress-related illnesses, and economic mobility.

The racial disparities in homeownership and neighborhood conditions are deeply rooted in barriers that keep African Americans in concentrated areas, coded for "away from whites." In the early 20th century, racially restrictive covenants were legal agreements embedded in property deeds that explicitly prohibited African Americans and other minorities from purchasing, leasing, or occupying homes in certain neighborhoods. These covenants were widespread, particularly during the 1920s and 1930s, and were used to maintain racial homogeneity in residential areas. They effectively confined African Americans to specific neighborhoods, limiting their access to quality housing, education, and economic opportunities. Although the Supreme Court declared these covenants unenforceable in 1948, their legacy has had a lasting impact on residential segregation.[101]

To add insult to injury, one of the most defining moments in housing inequities for African Americans was introduced through the enactment of redlining. A federally sanctioned policy that began in the 1930s involved the Home Owners' Loan Corporation (HOLC) and Federal Housing Administration (FHA) systematically categorizing Black neighborhoods as "high-risk" investment areas.[102] These designations meant that Black families were systematically denied access to mortgages, home loans, and federal housing subsidies, preventing them from purchasing homes or building generational wealth. Meanwhile, white communities were deemed "low-risk" and given preferential access to federal mortgage assistance, fostering suburban expansion and generational wealth-building. This practice not only determined who could purchase homes, but also dictated the allocation of resources for schools, infrastructure, and essential services. By 1968, when the Fair Housing Act was passed, nearly 98% of FHA-backed loans had gone to white families, locking Black communities into a cycle of disinvestment and generational poverty.[103]

The combined effect of racially restrictive covenants and redlining has had long-term consequences. These discriminatory practices reinforced residential segregation, leading to underinvestment in Black neighborhoods. This has resulted in disparities in education, healthcare, and employment opportunities that continue to affect African American communities today.[104] A study published in

Environmental Research Letters found that formerly redlined neighborhoods have higher rates of poverty, lower property values, and greater exposure to environmental hazards such as air pollution and lead contamination. These factors create a cascade of health risks, from respiratory illnesses to developmental disorders in children. In addition, studies have linked historical redlining to present-day health inequities that include higher rates of chronic diseases such as diabetes and hypertension in formerly redlined communities. The lack of investment in these areas has often meant limited access to healthcare facilities and healthy food options.[105] The deliberate acts of government-endorsed polices have cemented these transgenerational health disparities.

Despite the formal end of redlining, contemporary housing discrimination continues in more subtle but equally damaging ways. Black homeownership rates have remained stagnant for over 50 years, with more than a 29.3% deficit from equaling white homeownership as of 2022.[106] African Americans are also more likely to face loan denials or receive higher interest rates even when they have comparable creditworthiness to white applicants. Additionally, a growing body of research has revealed that Black homeowners often receive lower property appraisals, further limiting their ability to accumulate wealth through real estate[107] (Discussed further in the Socioeconomic Section).

Renters in Black communities also face higher eviction rates and unstable housing conditions. Studies show that Black women and children are disproportionately affected by eviction, a major driver of homelessness and economic insecurity.[108] The financial strain of eviction not only destabilizes families but also increases the risk of mental health conditions such as anxiety and depression. Housing instability is ranked as one of the highest social stressors. Research by David Williams highlights how social stressors like racial discrimination impact Black Americans' health, contributing to heightened cortisol levels from chronic stress.[109] Chapter 4 of this book outlines how this predisposes African Americans to an increased risk of hypertension, cardiovascular disease, and premature aging.

Another persistent challenge in housing for African Americans has been disinvestment in historically Black communities while simultaneously witnessing gentrification displace long-term Black residents. For decades, local governments and private investors have neglected the infrastructure, underfunded schools, and allowed the housing stock to deteriorate. In addition, the demise of public services and economic development in these areas exacerbated community conditions of poverty and isolation, while unemployment and crime rates increased. However, when these neighborhoods became desirable to wealthier, predominantly white residents, they experienced a sudden influx of investment, a process known as gentrification. Streets were repaved, new businesses opened, rent increased, and property values rose, often pricing out Black residents who had lived in these areas for generations. Between 2000 and 2013, nearly 135,000 Black residents were displaced from historically Black neighborhoods in major cities like Washington, D.C., New York, and San Francisco due to gentrification-driven housing costs.[110] The forced displacement erodes community cohesion and social networks, which are critical sources of mental and emotional well-being. Research has shown that being uprooted from one's community increases stress levels, exacerbates mental health challenges, and leads to weaker health outcomes in the long term.[111]

There is great value in community cohesion for fostering a sense of belonging. Black communities, which have historically relied on strong social networks for support and resilience, are fragmented as families are displaced. This loss of cohesion has significant health implications, as research indicates that social support and a sense of belonging are crucial for maintaining mental health and overall well-being.[112] When Black residents are forced to leave their neighborhoods, they lose not only their homes but also the churches, schools, and community centers that serve as anchors of identity and stability. Moreover, the influx of wealthier residents often leads to the erasure of Black cultural landmarks and institutions. For example, historic Black-owned businesses and cultural centers are replaced by cafes, upscale boutiques, and dog parks catering to white newcomers, further alienating the original residents. The loss of cultural and social landmarks during gentrification can create a psychological disconnection for displaced residents, which amplifies feelings of marginalization, loss of identity, and a sense of disconnection from what once was.[113] This displacement not only disrupts lives but also reinforces the message that Black communities are disposable, valued only when they can be monetized or appropriated.

Stable, safe, and affordable housing is a basic human right. Yet, its oppressive barriers serve as a foundation for keeping African Americans in a perpetual state of survival. The chronic stress of survival fueled by the combination of housing instability, forced displacement, and continued racialized barriers to homeownership exacerbates health disparities in the Black community. Affordability is key. Housing cost burden, where more than 30% of income is spent on rent or mortgage payments, disproportionately impacts Black families (55%) compared to white families (28%).[114] High housing costs force many to choose between rent and necessities like food, healthcare, and medications, exacerbating health disparities. Compounding this disparity is not limited to housing options alone. When residents are subjected to substandard housing conditions, including mold, lead exposure, inadequate insulation, and pest infestations, it contributes to higher rates of asthma, respiratory illnesses, and lead poisoning in Black children.[115] The cycle is vicious and only the tip of the iceberg as it relates to social determinants of health.

Dismantling Barriers: Addressing Housing Inequities

To address the housing-related health disparities faced by African Americans, policymakers must prioritize equitable and inclusive housing policies. That include:

1. **Reversing the legacy of redlining:** Invest in predominantly Black neighborhoods without the prerequisite of gentrification, ensuring that resources benefit the existing residents.

2. **Affordable housing initiatives:** Increase access to affordable housing options that enable families to remain in their communities while benefiting from revitalization efforts.

3. **Stronger tenant protections:** Enact policies to prevent displacement and provide rent stabilization for long-term residents.

An example of efforts that demonstrate barrier-breaking in housing initiatives includes:

The Douglass Community Land Trust (DCLT) in Washington, D.C. is a great example of a barrier-breaking housing initiative. This non-profit organization established in 2019 that focuses on creating and preserving affordable housing in areas at risk of gentrification. By acquiring land and ensuring it remains dedicated to affordable housing, the trust empowers residents to remain in their communities and benefit from neighborhood revitalization efforts without the threat of displacement.[116]

BARRIER TWO:
EDUCATION AS A GATEKEEPER TO OPPORTUNITY

Education is one of the most powerful social determinants of health, shaping opportunities, economic mobility, and access to essential resources. For African Americans, however, the education system in the United States has historically been and remains a tool for perpetuating systemic inequities. From underfunded schools and biased disciplinary practices to the lingering effects of segregation, the American education system has not only limited opportunities for Black students but also contributes to poor health outcomes that continue to persist. The inequities in education are not limited to curriculum or pedagogy; they extend to the very infrastructure of schools, the allocation of resources, and the implicit messages that

Black students receive about their value in society. For many Black children, the education system becomes a daily reinforcement of the structural inequities designed to oppress them.

The roots of educational inequities lie in the segregationist policies of the 19th and 20th centuries. Although the Brown v. Board of Education decision in 1954 declared school segregation unconstitutional, the legacy of segregation remains deeply embedded in the fabric of American education. Predominantly Black schools continue to face significant funding gaps, with schools in nonwhite districts receiving $23 billion less annually than their predominantly white counterparts, as reported by EdBuild in 2020.[117] The reliance on local property taxes to fund public schools perpetuates this disparity. Wealthier, predominantly white communities have access to better-funded schools with advanced resources, smaller class sizes, and plentiful extracurricular programs. In contrast, predominantly Black neighborhoods, shaped by redlining and economic disinvestment, are left with underfunded schools, outdated textbooks, and inadequate technology. This disparity not only limits academic opportunities for Black students but also reinforces the systemic undervaluation of their potential.

Overcrowded classrooms further exacerbate the problem. Teachers in these settings struggle to provide individualized attention, leaving many students behind. According to the National Assessment of Educational Progress, only 17% of Black fourth graders achieved reading proficiency in 2022, compared to 42% of white students.[118] This literacy gap has long-term consequences, especially when combined with living in poverty. African American children are overrepresented in both of these categories, therefore quadrupling their risk of dropping out of high school or not graduating on time.[119] Low literacy levels can ultimately limit career opportunities that perpetuate cycles of poverty and increase the risk of criminal justice system engagement. Statistics show that 85% of juveniles in the justice system are functionally illiterate, and 75% of the US prison population are high school dropouts.[120] This lends credence to African Americans being disproportionately incarcerated in comparison to their white counterparts.

Racial biases in disciplinary practices compound these challenges. Black students are three times more likely than white students to be suspended or expelled, according to the U.S. Department of Education, even for similar infractions. These harsh disciplinary actions further contribute to the school-to-prison pipeline, defined by sociologist Mark Warren as "an interlocking system of policies and practices that push students of color from low-income communities out of school and into the juvenile and criminal justice system. These policies and practices include exclusionary discipline (suspensions and expulsions) and increased policing."[121] Studies show that experiencing a suspension during grades 7-12 is significantly associated with greater odds of incarceration in young adulthood.[122] An uncorrected foundation of early academic failure creates student disengagement over time that can feed into a vicious cycle of behavioral problems perceived as disruptive, warranting a need for disciplinary actions. The entire Black community is left at a disadvantage when the lack of early interventions incapacitates the young, malleable minds of these students' ability to truly thrive in life.

The physical environment of schools attended by Black students often mirrors the inequities they experience in society. Dilapidated buildings with peeling paint, broken windows, and insufficient resources send an implicit message that Black children's education, and by extension, their futures, are not a priority. Substandard facilities not only affect academic performance but also reinforce a sense of inferiority among students. Jonathan Kozol points out in his book "The Shame of the Nation" how such disinvested academic environments can take a psychological toll by passively teaching Black children they are undeserving of the same opportunities as their white peers. This devaluation can become internalized, leading to a lack of self-worth, disinterest in learning, and a decline in aspirations.

Additionally, the lack of representation in curricula and among educators further marginalizes Black students. U.S. history textbooks often reduce Black history to slavery and civil rights, erasing the rich contributions of Black Americans in science, art, literature, and leadership. This exclusion denies Black students the opportunity to see themselves reflected in positions of excellence and influence beyond sports and entertainment, as seen in the media. Representation among educators is equally critical. Black teachers comprise only 7% of public-school educators, despite Black students making up 15% of the student population.[123] Research published in Educational Researcher shows that Black students with at least one Black teacher during elementary school are significantly more likely to graduate from high school and pursue higher education. The lack of Black educators denies students the mentorship and cultural understanding that can enhance their educational experiences.

For some Black students, pursuing quality education necessitates commuting beyond their local neighborhoods to attend better-resourced schools, often situated in predominantly white areas. This pursuit, while aimed at academic advancement, introduces additional challenges that can adversely affect health and well-being. Extended commute times require students to wake up earlier than usual, which reduces the essential sleep needed for physiological restoration and cognitive development. Research suggests that longer school commutes can have a negative impact on the physical and mental well-being of students.[124] Longer commutes equate to longer periods of being sedentary that can lead to obesity, and shorter time sleeping that can impair memory and mood, both of which can lead to pathways of students' health becoming diminished over time.

Moreover, the time spent commuting, sometimes up to three hours round trip, can also lessen opportunities for homework, extracurricular activities, and family engagement. This imbalance means that Black students enduring lengthy commutes are not afforded the same 24 hours as their white peers, who often attend local schools with much shorter commute times. The added stress also extends to parents, who may need to adjust work schedules or incur additional transportation costs. While accessing better educational opportunities is a commendable goal, the associated health and social costs ultimately can place these striving students at another disadvantage, adding to their cumulative health burden.

The desire to escape poverty is a powerful motivator that compels parents to make short-term sacrifices in terms of health and well-being for the long-term benefit of increased financial options for their children. Educational inequities are a significant driver of the cycle of poverty in Black communities. Students themselves are often hyper-aware of what is at stake. In Woods-Giscombe's study on African American women, "one young college student in particular discussed that her ambition and drive for success were related to others' expectations that she would fail in life because she was African American."

Without access to quality education, many Black students are funneled into low-wage jobs with limited benefits and opportunities for advancement. This economic instability forces families to adopt a survival-oriented mindset, prioritizing immediate needs over long-term goals. When school systems fail to provide Black students with the necessary tools and resources for success, Black pupils become conditioned to perpetuate a cycle of poverty that feeds into the social health determinant disparities. This cycle not only limits economic mobility but also entrenches survival as a way of life, leaving little room for investment in preventive health or personal development.

While students on the proverbial "Southside" may experience dilapidated buildings. High student-teacher ratios and potentially long commutes to out-of-area schools, Black students on the other side of the tracks, and the reality of stress hits them differently. More resources, particularly when obtained in predominantly white schools, come with their own set of problems that go by a different name, like implicit racial bias in subjective grading methods. Countless microaggressions, comprising subtle yet offensive comments, are frequently heard from both students and teachers. Experiences of these slights may sound petty, but one Black student describes it as "death by a thousand cuts." It's the allostatic load bearing the weight of compounded frustrations, anger, and downright disgust at times.

Feeling invisible or the need to compromise the identity of Blackness for the sake of fitting in and surviving the terrain is real pressure. During my first year at Princeton, a young African American freshman would come over regularly to our Seminary dining hall and eat with us graduate students as a way to engage with the Black community. He had locks in his hair, he appeared culturally connected, and he was gifted in African dance. Over time, he stopped coming around our small fellowship of Black students until I saw him at the end of the academic year. He had dropped his cultural cadence to sound more like his white peers and seemed to want to look more like them with his new blue contact lenses, despite his melanin-rich skin. I was deeply saddened for him, but understood the pressure of conformity in an environment where you are deemed as "other."

Therefore, the consequences of educational inequities extend far beyond the classroom, profoundly shaping health outcomes. Education influences income, employment, and access to healthcare, all of which are critical determinants of health. Individuals with lower levels of education are more likely to experience chronic illnesses such as hypertension, diabetes, and heart disease. Chronic stress (discussed in chapter 4) is a key driver of health disparities; it is often a byproduct of navigating an inequitable education system. Black students face racial biases from teachers and peers, leading to feelings of alienation and "stereotype threat," which is the risk of confirming negative stereotypes about one's racial group. In such instances, students are more focused on avoiding failure than on achieving success.[125] An academic journey paved with this type of chronic stress can contribute to mental health challenges, including anxiety and depression, which can persist into adulthood. The psychological toll of the various components of educational neglect also manifests in maladaptive coping mechanisms such as substance use, overeating, and disengagement from healthcare. These behaviors increase the risk of chronic diseases and further widen the health disparities between Black and white populations.

Dismantling Barriers: Equitable Education for All

To address these systemic inequities, a multifaceted approach is required:

1. **Equitable Resource Allocation**: Ensure that schools in Black communities receive the necessary funding for advanced coursework, extracurricular activities, and updated technology.

2. **Diverse Educator Recruitment:** Increase efforts to recruit and retain Black teachers to serve as role models and mentors for Black students.

3. **Disciplinary Reform:** Implement restorative justice practices to address racial disparities in school discipline.

An example of efforts that exemplify barrier-breaking in education initiatives includes:

Restorative Practices in Oakland Unified School District: OUSD has developed a restorative justice training program for educators to reduce racial disparities in school discipline. These practices are designed to replace strict disciplinary policies with a focus on building strong in-school relationships. OUSD's initial reported findings indicate that creating a greater sense of community within the schools has led to a reduction in absenteeism and dropout rates, while the reading levels have increased. There has also been a decrease in suspension rates, and "racially disproportionate discipline of African-American students eliminated in some of our (OUSD) schools."[126]

BARRIER THREE:
FOOD APARTHEID AND NUTRITIONAL ACCESS

Access to nutritious and affordable food is essential for health and well-being. Yet, African Americans disproportionately face barriers to accessing healthy foods, with systemic racism shaping the food environments in predominantly Black communities. These inequities are not isolated incidents but a continuation of historical patterns of neglect and devaluation, rooted in the systemic exploitation of Black bodies during slavery and perpetuated through contemporary practices. Food has become another tool used to create an inequitable distribution of one of the body's most essential resources: nutrition. Food injustice serves as a blatant reminder that Black health remains undervalued in the United States.

In Chapter 3, we explored how enslaved Africans were deliberately denied access to adequate nutrition, receiving meager rations that failed to meet their caloric and nutritional needs. This deprivation weakened their bodies, increased susceptibility to disease, and laid the groundwork for the chronic health disparities that persist today. Enslaved women, forced to sustain pregnancies and nurse their children on inadequate diets, passed these nutritional deficits to their offspring, creating a legacy of compromised health. Fast forward to the present day, and the systemic neglect of Black health continues in the form of food deserts and food swamps. This level of food injustice is disproportionately affecting predominantly Black neighborhoods. A study published in Health & Place found that the majority of Black and low-income neighborhoods have significantly fewer supermarkets and more fast-food outlets than predominantly white neighborhoods.[127] This disparity is not the result of random choices; it reflects decades of discriminatory practices such as redlining and retail redlining. Deliberate discriminatory zoning laws and historical exclusion of Black communities' economic development initiatives have hindered investments in grocery infrastructure. The magnitude of this disinvestment has left Black and Brown communities as the highest populations represented among the 20% of American households situated in food deserts—areas with scarce availability of grocery stores, farmers markets, and restaurants, all of which significantly restrict access to affordable and nutritious food choices.[128]

Limited access to full-service grocery stores in Black communities has created an over-reliance on more readily accessible substitutions offering high-calorie, nutrient-poor options, otherwise known as food swamps. A study in The Journal of Preventive Medicine revealed that neighborhoods with predominantly Black residents had 2.4 times more fast-food outlets per square mile than predominantly white neighborhoods.[129] Meanwhile, non-fast-food options most readily available are found in dollar stores and convenience stores, also over-saturating minority and low-income areas. These establishments predominantly offer heavily processed and packaged foods, often lacking essential nutrients in fresh produce and more wholesome options. The strategic influx of unhealthy food options reflects a deliberate neglect of Black health, perpetuating diet-related chronic conditions and widening health disparities. The abundance of calorie-dense, nutrient-depleted options in food swamps and deserts directly contributes to the high prevalence of obesity, diabetes, hypertension, and cardiovascular disease among African Americans. These conditions, deeply tied to diet, reflect the cumulative impact of systemic neglect on Black health.

The prevalence of food swamps and food deserts in Black communities is a stark indicator that the systemic devaluation of Black health has not ended but merely evolved. While enslaved bodies were once monetized through forced labor, the contemporary food system is yet another structural barrier ensuring that Black communities remain at a disadvantage, undermining their ability to thrive in well-being and success. Marginalization is further demonstrated in research indicating that low-income, high-percentage minority communities have a higher concentration of alcohol outlets compared to wealthier areas, providing a juxtaposition between accessibility to a 40 oz container of health-destructive alcohol being made easier than obtaining a pound of life-giving collard greens and sweet potatoes. The clustering of such outlets, coupled with the scarcity of grocery stores offering healthy food options, underscores systemic inequities that perpetuate health disparities in Black communities.

Sustainable nutrition is foundational to raising strong children to build strong communities. According to research by Dr. Deborah Frank, founder of the Grow Clinic for Children, food insecurity contributes to a condition known as growth faltering or failure to thrive, where children's physical growth and cognitive development are stunted due to inadequate nutrition. This circumstance, rooted in systemic neglect, affects entire communities, where the lack of nutritious food perpetuates cycles of poor health, low productivity, and economic instability. According to the U.S. Department of Agriculture Report, more than 20% of Black households are food insecure, compared to 7% of white households. Dr. Marion Nestle, a leading expert in food politics, discusses in her book *Food Politics: How the Food Industry Influences Nutrition and Health,* how the food environment is a reflection of power dynamics. A lack of vital resources, such as access to healthy foods in Black communities, speaks volumes about whose health is prioritized in our society and whose is not. Social opponents have stated that all lives matter, but driving across America's landscape of neighborhoods accurately depicts a strong visual of whole communities that undoubtedly do not matter to the powers that be.

The health consequences of systemic neglect in food access are severe, as seen in African Americans leading the nation in diet-related chronic conditions that include: Obesity, whereas, according to the CDC, African Americans are 1.5 times more likely to be obese in comparison to their white counterparts. Obesity is also a major risk factor for diabetes, hypertension, and heart disease. Statistics from the Department of Health and Human Services Office of Minority Health indicate that Black adults are 1.4 times more likely than white adults to be diagnosed with diabetes.[130] What is more devastating is that African Americans are nearly twice as likely to die from diabetes.

African Americans have the highest rates of hypertension, a condition exacerbated by high-sodium diets commonly found in food swamps. Not to mention, being diagnosed with any of these conditions can complicate pregnancy and delivery, adding to the burden of poor nutrition during pregnancy, therefore increasing the risk of preterm births and low birth weights, all conditions that disproportionately affect Black mothers, infants, and subsequent generations.

The psychological toll of food insecurity further exacerbates these health outcomes. The stress of not knowing where one's next meal will come from or being unable to consistently provide nutritious food for one's family contributes to chronic stress, anxiety, and depression. In addition, for children, food insecurity impairs cognitive development, academic performance, and social interactions, perpetuating cycles of disadvantage. Meanwhile, there is the added burden of stress associated with society disregarding the root cause of structural inequities that hinder access to nutritious foods while amplifying a narrative of poor individual behavioral and lifestyle choices of the Black community, creating this disease prevalence.

Dismantling the Barriers: Solutions for Food Equity

Key strategies to address food inequities in Black communities include:

1. **Policy Reforms**: Strengthen programs like SNAP and WIC to ensure food security for low-income families. Advocate for zoning reforms to incentivize grocery stores and farmers' markets in underserved neighborhoods.

2. **Environmental Justice**: Address the structural barriers that perpetuate food deserts and swamps, including discriminatory zoning laws and retail practices.

3. **Education and Advocacy**: Implement nutrition education programs in schools and communities to promote healthy eating habits and empower residents to demand equitable access to nutritious food.

PART II STRUCTURAL BARRIERS TO WELLNESS

An example of efforts that exemplify barrier-breaking food access initiatives includes:

Oasis Fresh Market in Tulsa, Oklahoma, opened its doors to the community in May 2021, marking the first Black-owned grocery store in Tulsa in over 50 years. This business directly addresses the food desert conditions in North Tulsa by providing residents with access to fresh produce, meats, and other essential groceries. Through forming partnerships with other local organizations, Oasis equips its residents with cooking classes and nutrition workshops that nurture healthier eating habits. They are not the average grocery store, but a refuge for the community to access resources to other vital needs beyond food that include housing, employment, health screenings, and other social services that promote economic empowerment and community revitalization.

BARRIER FOUR:
HEALTHCARE DENIAL, DELAY, AND DISMISSAL

Access to quality healthcare is a cornerstone of health and well-being, yet systemic racism has entrenched profound disparities in healthcare access and outcomes for African Americans. These inequities, deeply rooted in the historical exploitation of Black bodies, persist today in the form of underfunded healthcare facilities, provider biases, inadequate treatment, and delayed diagnoses. Together, these barriers undermine the health of Black communities, perpetuating cycles of mistrust, inequity, and preventable suffering. This creates a cumulative impact leading to increased stress, thereby worsening health disparities and reducing life expectancy for African Americans. Ultimately, research shows us that the lasting effects of these barriers contribute to the higher morbidity and mortality rates across various conditions while intensifying health risks for future generations.

The roots of healthcare inequities in Black communities stretch back to slavery, where the enslaved were denied basic medical care unless it served the economic interests of their enslavers. The dehumanization of Black bodies during this era was heightened by exploitation for medical experimentation, as seen in the infamous Tuskegee Study of Untreated Syphilis in the Negro Male. A government-facilitated study conducted from 1932 to 1972 involved 600 Black men who were misled into believing they were receiving free medical care, while treatment was deliberately withheld to study the progression of untreated syphilis. In addition, there was the non-consensual use of Henrietta Lacks' cells in scientific research. These cells became the HeLa cell line, instrumental in numerous medical breakthroughs, yet her family was neither informed nor compensated, exemplifying exploitation in medical research. These historical abuses, among many others, established a legacy of mistrust in the healthcare system, a suspicion that persists today in the Black community. This is evidenced in lower doctor-patient rapport when there is a racial discordance, and also in lower participation rates among Blacks in clinical trials and organ donations.

Following emancipation, systemic racism continued to shape healthcare access for African Americans. Segregationist policies relegated Black patients to underfunded and overcrowded hospitals that lacked adequate resources for proper care. A study highlighted that in the Southern United States, only 6% of hospitals offered unrestricted services to Black individuals, while 31% denied them admission entirely, and 47% maintained segregated wards.[131] To further the discrimination, the same segregationist policies blocked Black physicians and nurses from practicing in well-equipped hospitals, restricting their professional development, thereby reinforcing a cycle of inadequate care within Black communities. The disparity in care was not incidental but deliberate, ensuring that Black communities remained marginalized. This segregation persisted well into the 20th century, leaving a lasting impact on the structure of healthcare access. Daniel Dawes, in his book *The Political Determinants of Health*, discusses how the historical exclusion of African Americans from healthcare resources was not just a matter of neglect but a matter of public policy—political measures erected with inequitable policies strategically designed to marginalize and devalue Black lives.

Today, the remnants of historical injustices remain visible in the healthcare landscape as health insurance coverage remains a significant barrier to healthcare access for African Americans. Factoring in that they are less likely than white Americans to have access to preventive care, specialty services, and advanced treatments. According to the Kaiser Family Foundation, Black adults are nearly twice as likely as white adults to report lacking a usual source of care, and they are more likely to delay or forgo medical treatment due to cost. Despite improvements following the implementation of the Affordable Care Act (ACA), disparities persist. African Americans are overrepresented among the uninsured, with 10.8% of Black adults lacking health insurance in 2022 compared to 6.8% of white adults.[132] Employer-sponsored insurance is a primary source of health coverage in the United States; however, disparities in access to such benefits exist. As of 2019, 66% of white workers had employer-sponsored health insurance, compared to 47% of Black workers.[133] This discrepancy is partly due to occupational segregation, where Black workers are overrepresented in industries less likely to offer health benefits. The lack of insurance coverage among Black Americans leads to not only delays in seeking care but also reduced access to preventive services and, ultimately, poorer health outcomes. Without insurance, following up with appointments and medications becomes cost-prohibitive, causing health ailments to significantly reduce quality of life.

Geographic disparities also play a significant role. Healthcare facilities in predominantly Black neighborhoods, particularly in rural areas and inner cities, often face chronic underfunding, understaffing, and clinic shortages, leading to longer wait times and delays in accessing care. A 2021 report from the National Association of Community Health Centers revealed that health centers serving Black communities receive less funding per patient than those in predominantly white areas, despite serving populations with greater health needs. These delays can have devastating consequences. Early detection is critical for managing diseases such as cancer, diabetes, and cardiovascular conditions. Yet, Black patients are more likely to receive delayed diagnoses, which often result in advanced-stage diseases that are more difficult and expensive to treat. For example, breast cancer mortality rates are 40% higher for Black women than for white women, despite 5% lower incidence rates.[134] This disparity is partly driven by various factors that include higher obesity prevalence (a cancer risk factor), later stages of diagnosis, barriers to completing treatment, and a higher prevalence of more aggressive subtypes of breast cancer (triple-negative and inflammatory).

This scarcity of healthcare facilities is especially pronounced for specialized services such as maternal healthcare, contributing to the palpable disparities in maternal and infant mortality rates. A 2021 CDC report revealed that Black women are three times more likely than white women to die from pregnancy-related complications, regardless of income or education level. Notably, over 80% of these pregnancy-related deaths in the U.S. are preventable.[135] This stark disparity underscores systemic issues within healthcare that disproportionately affect Black women. Most notably, racial bias is highlighted as a key driver in this health gap.

Data shows that racial bias among healthcare providers is a significant barrier to equitable care and is undeniably harmful. Black patients often report that their concerns are dismissed or minimized, a pattern that erodes trust and undermines the doctor-patient relationship. A study published in JAMA Health Forum found that Black patients often felt that clinicians dismissed their concerns, including the severity of symptoms and pain levels, and provided inadequate information about medications and treatment plans. This dismissiveness contributed to feelings of skepticism toward the healthcare system.[136]

An eye-opening study indicating racial bias and its potential for detrimental impact was found in Proceedings of the National Academy of Sciences, which revealed that some medical trainees falsely believed that Black patients have thicker skin and less sensitive nerve endings than white patients.[137] These misconceptions lead to disparities in pain management, with Black patients less likely to receive pain medication for the same conditions as their white counterparts. As seen in emergency departments, Black patients with bone fractures are less likely to be administered pain medication compared to whites.[138] In a 2022 Pew Study on Health disparities, one woman described her husband's struggle with pain management: "My husband's condition... it requires a narcotic... for so long, a lot of people just assumed that he was a junkie, like he was just coming in and trying to get pain medication and they wanted to put him on this rotation that just didn't work, wanted him to take this Tylenol. And it was so frustrating."

The bias extends beyond pain management. Providers may second-guess the need for advanced diagnostics or treatments for Black patients, delaying critical interventions. For example, research indicates that Black patients presenting with cardiovascular symptoms are less likely to receive advanced diagnostic procedures and specialist consultations compared to their white counterparts. A study published in Circulation found that Black and Hispanic patients with congestive heart failure had 13% fewer follow-up consultations than white patients, even after adjusting for various factors.[139] Additionally, research reported in the Journal of the American College of Cardiology revealed that Black women were significantly less likely to be referred for cardiac catheterization than white men, with Black race negatively influencing the decision-making process for heart transplants.[140] These disparities highlight systemic biases in healthcare that contribute to unequal treatment outcomes for Black patients.

Disturbing studies reveal that 70% of physicians exhibit some level of implicit bias against Black and Hispanic/Latino patients, affecting diagnosis and treatment decisions.[141] These disparities in care delay health protection, thereby exacerbating disease progression and financial burden. A tragic example of this is Dr. Susan Moore, a

Black physician who, while battling COVID-19 in 2020, documented her experiences of inadequate care and dismissal of her pain by a white physician. She stated, "This is how Black people get killed, when you send them home, and they don't know how to fight for themselves."[142] Dr. Moore's subsequent death highlights the severe consequences of racial bias in medical treatment.

Dismantling the Barriers: Solutions for Equitable Healthcare

To dismantle the systemic barriers in healthcare, targeted interventions are needed:

1. **Implicit Bias Training**: Mandate comprehensive training programs for all healthcare educators and providers to address racial biases and improve cultural competence.
2. **Equitable Funding**: Increase funding for community health centers in predominantly Black neighborhoods to ensure timely access to quality care.
3. **Diverse Workforce Development**: Recruit and retain more Black healthcare providers and administrators to build trust and improve representation on all levels within the medical field.

An example of efforts that exemplify barrier-breaking health services access initiatives includes:

In September of 2024, the **United Kingdom's National Health Service** piloted a virtual reality training program to address racism and discrimination among its staff. Training materials incorporate findings from the TIDES study, whose goal is to understand how discrimination witnessed or experienced by healthcare practitioners contributes to inequalities in health service use. The actual training involves reenacted scenarios of workplace racism to foster empathy and improve responses to discrimination, with the aim of creating a more inclusive healthcare environment.[143]

PART II STRUCTURAL BARRIERS TO WELLNESS

BARRIER FIVE:
LABOR INEQUITY AND ECONOMIC FRAGILITY

Employment is the gateway to financial stability, access to healthcare, and a sense of purpose. Yet, systemic racism in the labor market creates persistent barriers for African Americans, resulting in higher unemployment rates, wage disparities, and occupational segregation. These inequities have profound consequences for physical, mental, and emotional well-being, perpetuating cycles of disadvantage and poor health.

Racial discrimination in hiring is a significant barrier for African Americans seeking equitable employment opportunities. Studies consistently show that Black job applicants face biases that limit their access to jobs. In a landmark study published in The American Economic Review (2004), Bertrand and Mullainathan submitted identical résumés with traditional-sounding names for Black and white Americans, respectively. Résumés with Black-sounding names, such as Jamal and Lakisha, were 50% less likely to receive callbacks than those with white-sounding names, such as Emily and Greg.[144] These biases stem from negative presumptions associated with Black-sounding names, including beliefs that applicants are less educated, less productive, less trustworthy, and less reliable. A follow-up study in the American Journal of Sociology added criminal records to the résumés of white-sounding names and found that white applicants with criminal records were called back for interviews at twice the rate of Black and Latino applicants without criminal backgrounds. These findings reveal how deeply ingrained racial biases continue to limit Black job seekers' baseline access to opportunities.

Workplace discrimination extends beyond hiring practices to the appearance of Black interviewees and employees. The pressure to conform to Eurocentric beauty standards often results in discriminatory practices against natural Black hairstyles, including afros, locs, braids, and twists worn by Black women and men. The 2023 CROWN Workplace Research Study showed that Black women are 2.5 times more likely than their white counterparts to have their hair perceived as unprofessional in the workplace. It also revealed that 54% of Black women feel they must straighten their hair to be considered successful during job interviews.[145] This pressure has led to the enactment of the Crown Act, a law prohibiting hair-based discrimination, which is now in effect in 23 states and jurisdictions around the United States. Without such protections, corporations often use something as trivial as hairstyles as another barrier to deny Black people access to upward mobility.

For those who succumb to the European standards of beauty, the trade-off comes with its associated health risk. Sitting in the beauty salon chair with a burning scalp once upon a time was a momentary sacrifice for the greater gain of more desirable and universally acceptable straight hair. However, science has revealed that there are alarming health costs associated with hair-straightening products. Studies indicate that chemical straighteners contain toxic endocrine disruptors, increasing the risk of hormone-sensitive cancers such as uterine and breast cancers.[146] This creates an added physical health burden to the psychological toll of conforming to discriminatory workplace standards. The hurdles are endless as one races towards survival in either economic sufficiency or better health; no one should have to choose. However, with each compounding barrier, society attempts to make thriving nearly impossible for African Americans.

Income is a must-have for economic survival; one must first get their foot in the door, and chronic stress ensues when that is repeatedly blocked. With livelihood at stake for many people, resources will be attained by any means necessary, as seen in the saturation of African Americans in low-wage service jobs, which can compound health risk factors. Many African Americans are employed in industries with high physical demands and low job security, further exacerbating stress and its associated health risks. For example, a study by the Economic Policy Institute (2020) found that Black workers are overrepresented in industries like food service and retail, where the risk of workplace injury and long hours is common.[147] Cross-cultural studies analysis indicates significant health risk factors associated with these low-ranking positions, and when racial discrimination is added into the equation, it only amplifies the problem.

The British Whitehall studies provide a valuable lens through which to examine the impact of workplace conditions on health. Conducted over several decades, these studies analyzed the health outcomes of British civil servants and uncovered a steep gradient in health outcomes based on occupational rank. The findings revealed that individuals in lower-ranking jobs experienced significantly worse health outcomes than their higher-ranking counterparts, even when accounting for lifestyle factors like smoking and exercise. One of the key findings from the first Whitehall study, published in The Lancet (1967), was that Individuals in the lowest employment grades were more than twice as likely to die prematurely from heart disease compared to individuals in the highest employment grades. The Whitehall II study, published in The Lancet (1991), built upon this by identifying the underlying causes: chronic stress, lack of job control, and perceived lack of respect in the workplace were all critical drivers of poor health outcomes.[148] Importantly, these disparities existed despite the universal healthcare system in the United Kingdom, highlighting that workplace conditions themselves were a primary factor. Some of the findings from the Whitehall study II more specifically indicated that due to the stress of low job control and poor working conditions, the lowest occupational grade workers experienced significantly higher rates of heart disease and metabolic disturbances, contributing to conditions like obesity and insulin resistance.

The lessons of the Whitehall studies highlight the profound impact of workplace conditions on health. For African Americans in the United States, the situation is compounded by systemic racism and occupational segregation. Similar to the findings in the Whitehall studies, African Americans in low-wage, low-status jobs face chronic stress and a lack of autonomy, which contribute to disproportionately high rates of hypertension, diabetes, and other stress-related diseases. This situation lends credence to the higher prevalence rates of these conditions observed in the Black community. Chronic stress from low-status jobs, compounded by systemic barriers, is a recipe for disease vulnerabilities among African Americans.

In my own clinical experience, I provide health screenings at various businesses throughout the states of Georgia and South Carolina. Depending on the company I was contracting with that sent me to the site, I was either responsible for conducting a health screen (blood pressure, finger prick for blood workup, height, and weight) on a set number of individuals as part of a team, or I was solely responsible for briefly discussing the screening results with at least half or all participants. Nonetheless, I witnessed hundreds upon hundreds of case examples of how the work environment, inclusive of types of work, hours, and work culture, effected the employees. I mentally collected data and brief stories of why their blood pressure was elevated, in addition to other metabolic markers such as cholesterol, weight, and glucose levels exceeding normal ranges. I saw distinct differences between the overall metabolic factors of primarily white educators and administrators at high schools that looked like well-resourced college campuses vs. predominantly African American workers at a downtown county courthouse. I also noticed the differences between lab markers in the staff in high-rise corporate buildings on the affluent side of town versus the factory workers or prison staff in more rural areas adjacent to the city. Without fail, employee after employee spoke to me about the stress of the job, and it showed in their metabolic data. I saw with my own eyes resemblances of the British Whitehall studies come to life in the American South.

The unique lived experiences of Black people in higher-ranking positions can present similar health challenges as those found in low-ranking jobs, with stress playing a central role. Black executives may not be on their feet all day, but they find themselves on high alert from the perpetual pressure to overperform and overdeliver, only to be recognized as "half as good" as their white colleagues. In an intersectional exploration on Being Black in Corporate America, studies found that two-thirds of black professionals have to work harder than their colleagues to advance in their careers. One participant commented that, "I was raised by a single mother, and she would always say, "Don't be late, don't bring your problems to work, dress a certain way. Because we're Black, you've got to work harder than the others."[149] While African American professionals are not being degraded by rude customers that service workers frequently encounter, they do find themselves under the scrutiny of clients unwilling to overlook minor errors and therefore are not afforded the benefit of the doubt.

Lack of diverse representation in white dominant spaces subjects Black professionals to continuously interfacing with bureaucracies where they may be met with resistance to their presence and/or their voice. Such encounters show up in the form of microaggressions, often leaving them feeling overlooked and undervalued. Contributing to higher rates of racial prejudice experienced by Blacks in comparison to other races. One micro build-up after another creates a macro problem, as reported by one female executive. "If you walked over and poked someone on the shoulder, it would be mildly annoying. If you walked over and poked them on the shoulder in the same spot every day for thirty years, you would poke them on the shoulder one more time, and they would go nuts."[150] Disappointingly so, uniforms replaced by designer suits and briefcases do not serve as shields of protection from the myriad of ways that stress infiltrates the experience of Black people working in white spaces.

Types of positions are only one variable among many that serve as an employment stressor. Pay rate disparities further highlight workplace inequities. NEA Research analysis from census data determined that although there has been a significant increase in Black college graduates since 1980, there has not been a similar surge in earnings. The average rate of pay for Black men ($52,000) and Black women ($45,000) in 2020 was below the mean earnings (even when adjusting for inflation) of what white men were earning in 1980 ($53,000), which rose to $73,000 in 2020.[151] In 2021, the median weekly earnings for Black full-time workers were $806, compared to $1,064 for white workers, according to the Economic Policy Institute. This wage gap persists even when controlling for education, occupation, and experience. For example, Black college graduates earn approximately 20% less than their white counterparts.[152] Moreover, Black women face an additional layer of disparity, earning just 63 cents for every dollar earned by white, non-Hispanic men, according to the National Partnership for Women and Families.

During a journey of financial survival, the only thing worse than a low-paying, or thankless job, is no job. Limited work access also shows up in the unemployment rate for African Americans, which has consistently been higher than that of white Americans, reflecting deeply entrenched systemic inequalities. According to the U.S. Bureau of Labor Statistics, as of 2022, the unemployment rate for Black Americans was 6.2%, nearly double that of white Americans at 3.1%. This disparity is not a new experience; historical data reveal that the unemployment rate for African Americans has been roughly twice as high as that of whites for decades. Structural barriers, including discrimination in hiring practices, unequal access to quality education, and geographic segregation, all of which have been discussed, contribute significantly to these disparities.

The struggle is real for many African Americans in the quest for not only survival, but economic stratification. Everything about the capacity to maintain any person's livelihood is easily translated to financial resources. Therefore, the barriers that prevent anyone from utilizing their intellect, gifts, talents, and skills in exchange for needed resources can be a baseline driver of chronic stress. The physical and mental toll is amplified among African Americans while navigating the racial oppression embedded into a stackable barrier often disguised as only one.

Limited employment options restrict financial mobility and take a severe toll on psychological well-being. Employment is tied to a sense of purpose, identity, and self-worth. When African Americans are systematically excluded from equitable job opportunities or relegated to low-paying positions, it fosters feelings of inadequacy, defeat, and disconnection. A study in Social Science & Medicine (2016) found that individuals who feel undervalued at work are more likely to experience depression and anxiety. Not to mention, the systemic denial of opportunities can fracture one's sense of self, reinforcing internalized oppression and limiting aspirations. This defeated internal narrative adds to the cycle of stress and maladaptive coping strategies that include substance abuse, overeating, and other unhealthy behaviors.

Employment is far more than a means of earning a living; it is a critical determinant of health and well-being, as pointed out by researcher David Williams in his extensive studies on discrimination and health. For African Americans, systemic barriers in the labor market–ranging from hiring discrimination to pressures to conform to Eurocentric norms compound the challenges of achieving equity. These inequities are not incidental but deliberate, reflecting the broader societal structures designed to marginalize Black lives. The cycle of economic instability undermines upward mobility efforts, creating a circular relationship where financial insecurity reinforces health disparities and poor health further limits employment opportunities. All of which creates more extensive patterns of systemic inequities that comprise the whole wellness of the Black community.

Dismantling Barriers to Employment Equity

1. **Workplace Equity Training**: Mandate implicit bias and cultural competence training for hiring managers and executives to address workplace discrimination.

2. **Expanded Workforce Development**: Provide job training and apprenticeship programs that prepare African Americans for high-demand, high-paying industries.

3. **Living Wage Legislation**: Advocate for minimum wage policies that provide a livable income for all workers, particularly those in low-wage sectors.

An example of efforts that exemplify barrier-breaking employment access initiatives includes:

The National Black Worker Centers (NBWC) is working to reduce racialized outcomes in the labor market while improving economic impact. This organization connects a network of eleven Black Worker Centers across the US, focusing on issues affecting Black working people in their communities. These centers provide workforce development programs, advocate for fair employment practices, and work to dismantle systemic barriers to employment equity. By focusing on Black workers' unique challenges, NBWC plays a crucial role in promoting equitable employment opportunities.[153]

BARRIER SIX:
SOCIOECONOMIC DISADVANTAGE

Socioeconomic status (SES), encompassing income, wealth, education, and occupational prestige, is a critical determinant of health. For African Americans, systemic barriers rooted in the nation's history of slavery and ongoing structural racism have entrenched enormous SES disparities. These disparities perpetuate cycles of economic disadvantage and contribute to the pronounced health inequities that continue to plague Black communities.

The economic foundation of the United States was built on the backs of enslaved people of African ancestry. During the period of enslavement, the unpaid labor of millions of Black men, women, and children generated a contemporary comparison of trillions of dollars in wealth for slaveholding whites. According to the state of California's 2022 Reparation Task Force Report, the present-day equivalent of unpaid wages to enslaved individuals is estimated at over $14 trillion.[154] A phenomenal return on investment, unlike any other known to humankind. This wealth fueled the nation's economic success, building infrastructure such as agricultural fields, roads, and burgeoning industries, while creating generational wealth for white families and their descendants. Meanwhile, enslaved Blacks were denied the opportunity to accumulate wealth for themselves or their descendants. The legal and economic systems ensured their exploitation and dehumanization, leaving an economic gap that remains one of the most striking legacies of slavery.

The abolition of slavery in 1865 did not usher in economic freedom for African Americans. Unlike indentured servants (a servitude system that was soon replaced by the influx of enslaved Africans), who were given acres of land, a gun, a cow, and clothing after fulfilling their relatively shorter-term labor contracts, freed Blacks never received their 40 acres and a mule. Instead, they were released into a new reality of no infrastructure in place to help them thrive. To economically remind them that their inferior social status had not changed after centuries of enslavement, they were not only denied any reestablishment assets but, in contrast, were forced into a system of indebtedness to their former masters. A strategy known as sharecropping had arisen to keep them systematically oppressed. Under this exploitative system, Black families worked land owned by white farmers in exchange for a portion of the crops. However, the high costs of tools, seeds, and living expenses were deducted from their earnings, leaving them with little, if any, to live off of, let alone save. This debt cycle ensured that economic mobility remained out of reach. They went from having nothing to even that which they would earn in the future would still be owed to their former enslaver, keeping many of them in a perpetual cycle of debt.

In addition, the Black Codes were quickly established in 1865, which were laws designed to restrict the activities and freedoms of African Americans by criminalizing basic behaviors, such as loitering or not having proof of employment. Violating these laws often led to imprisonment, where African Americans were reintroduced to forced free labor under the convict leasing system. This was the precursor to today's prison-industrial complex, which ensured that free labor continued, disproportionately affecting Black men and ultimately their families, who lost them as a financial contributor to the household.

Even after the abolition of Black Codes in 1866, systemic barriers persisted. The Jim Crow era (1877-1968) reinforced segregation and restricted access to education, employment, housing, and other services for African Americans. The exclusion of Black Americans from New Deal programs was strategically implemented to hinder social stratification. This entailed excluding Domestic and agricultural workers, professions largely occupied by Black Americans, from the initial Social Security Act of 1935. In addition, Black veterans encountered discriminatory practices when they were routinely denied the GI Bill to access education, housing, and business loans, while white veterans used it to build economic success for themselves and their families. These barriers created an enduring wealth gap. Today, the median wealth of white families is nearly eight times that of Black families ($188,200 compared to $24,100, according to the Federal Reserve).[155] This disparity is a direct result of centuries of systemic economic oppression that continues to hold this gap in place, making it impossible to close without extraordinary means.

Homeownership is the primary vehicle for building generational wealth in the United States. Yet, it has been methodically denied to African Americans through decades of inequitable policies and practices. As of 2022, the Black homeownership rate in the United States was 45.3%, compared to 74.6% for white Americans, according to the U.S. Census Bureau. This stark disparity reflects the lingering impact of historical barriers such as redlining, racially restrictive covenants, and exclusion from the previously mentioned government programs. Wealth accumulation is primarily attained via homeownership; however, African Americans have been systematically excluded from this opportunity, hindering the ability to pass on financial stability to future generations.

The 2008 housing crisis further exacerbated these inequalities. Predatory lending practices disproportionately targeted Black borrowers, steering them toward subprime loans even when they qualified for more favorable terms. A study by the Center for Responsible Lending found that Black and Latino homeowners were twice as likely as white homeowners to experience foreclosure during the crisis. The loss of homes not only stripped families of their primary asset but also had long-term consequences for wealth accumulation and neighborhood stability.

Today, it's the same game with new barriers as Black homeowners contend with racial bias in home appraisals. Even when attaining the American Dream, Blacks continue to be placed at a further economic disadvantage compared to their white counterparts. Alarming results were revealed in a groundbreaking mystery-shopper testing in home appraisals conducted by the National Community Reinvestment Coalition. Findings included appraisers undervaluing homes they perceived were occupied by African Americans, 9-12.9% lower than when the same home was presented by a perceived white owner. Another study by the Brookings Institution in 2021 found that homes in Black neighborhoods are valued at 23% less than comparable homes in white neighborhoods, costing Black homeowners an average of at least $48,000 per home.[156] Undervalued appraisals can impact not only home selling price but also refinancing options and asset leverage towards other investments. After Black families jump over the hurdles to homeownership, they are later met with compounding barriers that deny them the opportunity to gain additional capital from it.

Living in a capitalist society where financial success equates to freedom and opportunity exacerbates the psychological burden of SES disparities for African Americans. The response to the depth of this burden can be summed up by the late R&B singer Marvin Gaye as he laments, "make me wanna holler and throw up both my hands." Witnessing the economic mobility of white Americans and other racial groups while being forced into a cycle of survival undoubtedly can foster feelings of frustration, inadequacy, and hopelessness. To be Black in America is to be assigned, upon birth, a barrier to thrive, only to break down those barriers and be met with new and more sophisticated obstacles repurposed under a different name. The resilience needed to not only build but maintain a successful life despite deliberate challenges comes at an emotional cost that can lead to chronic stress, depression, and previously discussed maladaptive coping mechanisms, all of which can further worsen health disparities.

For those who have not been able to be as successful with their resiliency, they still invest an enormous amount of time and energy to merely survive, with the mere hope of escaping the cycle of poverty one day. African Americans often work multiple jobs to make ends meet, leaving little room for personal development, community involvement, or health-promoting activities. Low SES also limits access to nutritious food, safe housing, and quality healthcare, all of which are individually and collectively critical for maintaining health. Financial insecurity, coupled with the psychological toll of systemic racism, again creates a feedback loop where these chronic stressors can accelerate biological aging and increase vulnerability to chronic disease.

The socioeconomic disparities faced by African Americans are not incidental but are the result of deliberate policies and practices designed to maintain racial hierarchies. These inequities not only limit economic mobility but also have profound implications for health and well-being. Currency is what creates access to all that is necessary to build and grow within the environment. Without addressing the wealth gap, it creates a further gap in disparities among all other resources, also sustained by currency.

Dismantling Socioeconomic Barriers

1. **Reparations**: Direct financial compensation for the descendants of enslaved African Americans to address the wealth gap created by slavery and systemic racism.

2. **Homeownership Support**: Policies that combat housing discrimination, provide down payment assistance, and ensure fair appraisals for Black homeowners.

3. **Workforce Equity**: Expanding access to high-paying jobs through education, training programs, and anti-discrimination enforcement.

An example of efforts that exemplify barrier-breaking socioeconomic access initiatives includes:

The City of Evanston, Illinois, became the first in the U.S. to implement a reparations program aimed at addressing the lasting socioeconomic impacts of slavery and discriminatory housing practices on Black residents. Funded by a $10 million commitment from cannabis tax revenue, the program provides up to $25,000 in housing assistance, including down payments, mortgage support, and home repairs to eligible Black residents or their descendants who lived in Evanston between 1919 and 1969. By directly investing in Black homeownership, Evanston's initiative serves as a model for addressing the racial wealth gap through local reparative justice.[157]

BARRIER SEVEN:
ENVIRONMENTAL RACISM AND TOXIC EXPOSURES

Environmental exposures significantly influence health, with systemic racism ensuring that African Americans bear a disproportionate burden of environmental hazards. These exposures, ranging from polluted air and water due to proximity to industrial sites, are not accidental. They are the result of deliberate decisions rooted in systemic racism, often referred to as environmental racism, which has perpetuated health disparities across generations.

Environmental racism is not a new trend. The placement of toxic waste facilities, industrial plants, and hazardous landfills has historically been concentrated in predominantly Black communities. This pattern was not incidental but intentional, rooted in a legacy of devaluing Black lives and property. Harriet A. Washington, in her groundbreaking book A Terrible Thing to Waste: Environmental Racism and Its Assault on the American Mind (2019), outlines how these practices have systematically exposed African Americans to environmental hazards, contributing to generational health inequities. For example, during the mid-20th century, urban renewal projects often displaced Black communities, pushing them into areas near industrial zones with high pollution levels. These areas became environmental sacrifice zones, where residents faced chronic exposure to pollutants that increased their risk of respiratory diseases, cancer, and other health conditions.

The Flint water crisis is one of the most egregious examples of environmental racism in recent history. In 2014, to save money, Flint officials switched the city's water supply from Lake Huron to the Flint River, a body of water known for its high levels of contamination. Corrosion inhibitors were not properly added to the water, causing lead to leach from aging pipes into the drinking water supply. The health impact of lead exposure, especially among Flint's predominantly Black population, has been catastrophic. Lead exposure is particularly harmful to children, causing irreversible brain damage, lower IQs, developmental delays, and behavioral problems. A 2018 JAMA Pediatrics study revealed a significant increase in blood lead levels among Flint's children following the water crisis. There has also been an increase in infant mortality rates, as indicated in a study published in Environmental Research, which found that fertility rates dropped by 12% and fetal death rates increased by 58% in Flint during the crisis.[158] The crisis persisted for over a year before any action was taken, despite residents' complaints and visible signs of water contamination. This neglect reflects a broader pattern of systemic disregard for Black communities' health and well-being.

In rural Black communities, particularly in the South, they face additional water contamination risks from agricultural runoff. This occurs when rainwater carries pesticides, fertilizers, and animal waste from farms into local water supplies. Agricultural runoff often contains high levels of nitrates, which can cause methemoglobinemia, or "blue baby syndrome," a condition that reduces the oxygen-carrying capacity of the blood. A study by the Environmental Working Group (2020) found that nitrate contamination disproportionately affects

PART II STRUCTURAL BARRIERS TO WELLNESS

rural communities with limited water treatment infrastructure, many of which are predominantly Black, Brown, Indigenous, or low-income communities. Residents living within 3 miles of these animal farms have also experienced respiratory ailments and a diminished quality of life from 10 billion gallons of fecal waste from pig farms being dumped in the nearby lagoon, impacting both the water and air supply.[159] This is seen specifically in North Carolina, where the number of pigs on farms is equivalent to three-quarters of the total state population of people. Poor rural areas are prime real estate for agricultural corporations to not only purchase cheap land, they also conduct business with limited accountability and value on the lives of the surrounding community. Neighboring residents within a few short miles of these facilities lack the individual and collective financial bandwidth needed to legally resist the environmental hazards introduced by these large corporations.

Whether in rural or urban areas, environmental pollution seems to be inescapable. African Americans are disproportionately exposed to air pollution due to the placement of truck depots, industrial plants, and petrochemical facilities in or near their communities. A 2019 study published in The Proceedings of the National Academy of Sciences found that African Americans are exposed to 56% MORE fine particulate matter (PM2.5) than they generate, compared to white Americans, who are exposed to 17% LESS than they create. Another study evaluating air pollution reveals even more stark findings in a steep incline of PM2.5 concentration seen in zip codes where African Americans make up more than 85% of the population.[160] The American Lung Association indicates that particulate matter pollution causes an increased risk of premature death among African Americans in comparison to white communities. At the same time, another study suggested that Blacks with higher incomes than whites still faced greater risk from air pollution, possibly due to the chronic stress of racial oppression.[161] In the lived experience of African Americans, it is all connected; all roads seem to lead back to compounded factors of chronic stress and multivariable injustices.

The pervasiveness of anti-Black racism still leaves the Black community vulnerable to disease when exposed to the social determinants of health.

Nonetheless, nowhere is the impact of industrial air pollution more apparent than in Cancer Alley, an 85-mile stretch of land along the Mississippi River where it sits between Baton Rouge and New Orleans, Louisiana. This area, home to more than 150 petrochemical plants and refineries, is predominantly Black and has some of the highest cancer rates in the country. According to the EPA, residents of Cancer Alley are 50 times more likely to develop cancer than the average American due to toxic air emissions. Particularly, residents of St. John the Baptist Parish, located in Cancer Alley, face cancer risks more than 800 times the national average due to emissions from nearby plants.[162] In addition, high levels of benzene and other volatile organic compounds in the air contribute to chronic respiratory conditions such as asthma and bronchitis. This toxic legacy illustrates how industrial zoning decisions prioritize profit over the health of Black communities, perpetuating a cycle of environmental and health inequities. One may argue that these plants bring life-sustaining employment opportunities to the area for some families; nonetheless, they still simultaneously jeopardize the lives of many who reside there and choose not to work at the plants.

Kat Stafford's piece on Black children with asthma features the horrifying phrase "I can't breathe, I can't breathe" from a child having an asthma attack.[163] This would cause any mother to be emotionally distressed, just as interviewee Catherine was, as she witnessed her terrified 5-year-old son clutch his small chest while continuously muttering these words. One would imagine her sense of panic when she discovered his inhaler was in the car and not on her person. Five-year-old Carter is among the 12% of Black children who suffer from this disease. Although it is manageable with routine appointments and inhalers, a larger percentage of Black children, in comparison to their white counterparts, end up in the emergency room in need of treatment. Unfortunately, a primary driver in this scenario, like many others, is the overlap between poverty and pollutants both inside and outside of the home, whereas "4 in 10 Black children live in areas with poor environmental and health conditions compared with 1 in 10 white children." Substandard affordable housing, exposing families to asthma triggers like dust and mold, gets compounded with nearby landfills, factories, and heavy emissions circulating in the air. All of which contributes to higher asthma mortality rates among Black children.

For Catherine, being the mom of two children with asthma propels additional stressors when the disease causes them to miss multiple school days and assignments, while she or their father is forced to miss work, leading to reduced household income. The burden of stress is internalized as Catherine states, "I'm the parent, the teacher, the nurse. It feels like you're kind of failing them." It is disappointing that her sense of defeat gets validated instead of consoled by the dominant society, as Kamora Herrington openly points out in the same article. "As a Black woman who is also a Black mother, I have experienced ridiculous amounts of blame and abuse from a larger system that understands they're culpable but understands that the issues are so big, that it's a whole lot easier to say, 'Black mommy, you're the problem." Black children are suffering from the multi-dimensional vulnerabilities of what it means to grow up impoverished and encounter a myriad of life-taking experiences that far outweigh life elements designed to cultivate their ability to thrive.

Global warming is impacting all beings everywhere, leaving Black communities at a greater disadvantage. The compounded effects of climate change exacerbate environmental injustices, particularly in historically redlined neighborhoods, many of which are predominantly Black. Urban heat islands, seen in urban areas with elevated temperatures due to dense development and limited greenery, are disproportionately located in these communities. A 2020 study analyzing 108 U.S. urban areas found that formerly redlined neighborhoods are, on average, 4.5°F hotter than non-redlined areas, with some cities experiencing temperature differences up to 12.6°F.[164] This significant temperature disparity arises from historical discriminatory housing policies that led to disinvestment in infrastructure and green spaces in these neighborhoods. The lack of tree canopy and the prevalence of heat-absorbing surfaces, such as asphalt and concrete, contribute to the intensified heat. Elevated temperatures increase the risk of heat-related illnesses, including heat stroke and exacerbation of cardiovascular and respiratory conditions. A study published in Environmental Health Perspectives highlighted that residents in formerly redlined areas face higher exposure to extreme heat, correlating with increased emergency department visits for heat-related issues.[165]

The disproportionate burden of environmental exposures among Black communities represents a significant yet often overlooked barrier to health, reinforcing systemic inequities that drive adverse health outcomes. From elevated levels of air pollution in predominantly Black neighborhoods to the legacy of toxic waste sites and inadequate access to clean water, these injustices are deeply rooted in structural racism and economic disinvestment. Chronic exposure to environmental hazards contributes to higher rates of respiratory illnesses, cardiovascular diseases, and other chronic conditions, exacerbating health disparities already shaped by socioeconomic and healthcare inequities. Harriet A. Washington skillfully demonstrates in *A Terrible Thing to Waste* just how deeply environmental racism penetrates far beyond pollutants but stretches into the systemic denial of humanity and dignity of communities of color. The ubiquitous nature of toxins and their contribution to the structural violence of their pervasive concentration in Black communities devalues the health and livelihood of residents with every breath.

Dismantling Environmental Racism
1. **Equitable distribution of Landfill Waste**: Reallocate landfill distribution centers so that they are not largely concentrated in Black areas.

PART II STRUCTURAL BARRIERS TO WELLNESS

2. **Stronger Regulations**: Enforce stricter environmental protections and penalties for industries that disproportionately pollute Black neighborhoods.
3. **Invest in Infrastructure**: Allocate funds to improve water and air quality in underserved communities, including updating aging pipes and reducing emissions near residential areas.

An example of efforts that exemplify barrier-breaking environmental racism initiatives includes:

Federal Investments in Safe Drinking Water Infrastructure: The Infrastructure Investment and Jobs Act (IIJA) allocated $50 billion to enhance drinking water infrastructure, with a focus on replacing lead service lines and ensuring safe water in underserved communities. This investment is particularly significant for Black communities that have historically faced challenges related to contaminated water supplies.[166]

BARRIER EIGHT:
SAFETY AND SURVEILLANCE

Public safety or the lack thereof shows up as another reminder for Black communities that their livelihood and well-being are not valued. The modern police force operates under the mandate to "protect and serve," yet for many African Americans, the presence of law enforcement does more to evoke fear and unease rather than safety. This tension stems from a historical and contemporary pattern of over-policing, racial profiling, and excessive use of force, which have eroded trust and created barriers to feeling secure in the presence of officers. Meanwhile, Black neighborhoods face infrastructure deficiencies that actively compromise health and safety rather than promoting it.

The origins of law enforcement in the United States are closely tied to the control and oppression of African Americans. During slavery, patrols were established to monitor and capture enslaved people who attempted to escape. After emancipation, these patrols evolved into formal police forces, tasked with enforcing Black Codes and later Jim Crow laws. These early forms of policing were explicitly designed to maintain racial hierarchies and economic exploitation, as Michelle Alexander highlights in *The New Jim Crow: Mass Incarceration in the Age of Colorblindness,* how the history of policing in the United States is inseparable from the history of racial oppression. The legacy of racial control persists in modern law enforcement practices. African Americans are disproportionately targeted by police, facing higher rates of stops, arrests, and use of force compared to their white counterparts. Data from the NYPD revealed that between 2002 and 2019, 83% of individuals stopped under stop-and-frisk policies were Black and Latino, despite these groups comprising only half of the city's population.[167] These encounters often escalate into violent interactions, contributing to a pervasive sense of fear and mistrust among African Americans.

According to a 2020 study in The Lancet, Black Americans are 2.5 times more likely to be killed by police than white Americans. This violence is not limited to high-profile cases but reflects a broader pattern of systemic discrimination. In addition, there is a negative health consequence beyond individuals directly involved, spilling over into the Black community at large. Research has demonstrated that police killings of unarmed Black individuals have adverse effects on the mental health of Black communities. In a study analyzing data from 2013 to 2015, it was found that each additional police killing of an unarmed Black person in a state was associated with an increase of approximately 0.14 poor mental health days among Black residents in the subsequent three months.[168] This effect was not observed when the individual killed was armed. These findings suggest that the perceived injustice and heightened sense of vulnerability following such incidents contribute to the mental distress experienced by Black communities. With every occurrence of these incidents, it perpetuates a stronger feeling of encounters with police representing violence instead of protection. This can take a psychological toll, contributing to chronic stress and mental health disorders such as PTSD and anxiety.

Barriers to feeling safe in the "Blue" Presence are evident in racial profiling and over-policing of Black bodies. Black people (men more specifically) are disproportionately stopped, searched, and surveilled by police. This creates a sense of hypervisibility that can make ordinary activities, like walking through one's own neighborhood, feel unsafe. According to data from the Bureau of Justice Statistics (2018), Black drivers are 20% more likely to be pulled over than white drivers, often without clear justification. Police Brutality, as seen in high-profile cases of police violence, such as the murders of George Floyd, Breonna Taylor, and countless others, also serves as a stark reminder of the potential for fatal outcomes during encounters with law enforcement. Cases such as these exacerbate distrust when the perception is that officers involved in misconduct often escape professional and/or legal accountability. A study by the Police Integrity Research Group at Bowling Green State University found that less than 2% of officers who killed civilians while on duty were charged with a crime, meaning 98.2% faced no legal action.[169] Further analysis by NPR revealed that in over 80 cases of fatal police shootings of unarmed Black people, authorities failed to charge the officers involved.[170] Of the few cases where charges were brought, only a small fraction resulted in convictions.

In addition to police surveillance, African Americans also have to deal with the stress of being under surveillance by white passersby. During slavery, to ensure the enslaved stayed "in their place" of subjugation, all white people were instructed to report any suspicious behavior of Black people. Although slavery ended in 1865, the community surveillance on Blacks continued around the country, with white people feeling entitled to know and question the presence and general activity of Black people and reporting their perceived suspicions to the police. Racially biased emergency calls often weaponize law enforcement against Black people engaged in everyday activities in public spaces. Spaces like barbecuing at the park, falling asleep while studying in the college student lounge, and sitting in Starbucks waiting for business associates before placing an order. Present-day social media outlets have played a significant role in polarizing these incidents of discrimination in hopes of reducing their long-standing occurrences. In an effort to deter these non-emergency discriminatory calls, there have been legislative initiatives implemented or considered in some states to make it unlawful, modeled after The CAREN's (Caution Against Racially Exploitative Non-Emergencies) Act, first introduced in San Francisco, California. Not feeling safe to freely exist in ALL spaces, not just some, becomes emotionally stressful and downright exhausting, as explained by Mary-Frances Winters in *Black Fatigue: How Racism Erodes the Mind, Body, and Spirit.*

The omnipresence of law enforcement in Black neighborhoods and Black events can create a militarized atmosphere, where residents feel policed rather than protected. This undermines community cohesion and increases stress, anxiety, and feelings of disenfranchisement. As sociologist Nikki Jones displays in *The Chosen Ones: Black Men and the Politics of Redemption,* the very system that purports to keep communities safe often perpetuates cycles of harm, particularly in Black communities. All of which directly or indirectly impacts the health disparities far beyond individuals directly involved in the encounters. This is seen not only when excessive use of force by police results in injuries and fatalities that disproportionately affect African Americans, but also the very fear of encountering the police for any reason is a source of chronic stress.

In addition to police encounters fostering a greater feeling of stress rather than safety, the physical environment is another critical but often overlooked dimension of public safety. The disinvestment in predominantly Black neighborhoods has created unsafe and poorly maintained infrastructures that limit opportunities for physical activity and social interaction, further exacerbating health disparities. In predominantly white neighborhoods, well-maintained infrastructure supports active lifestyles through amenities such as bike lanes, walking trails, and attractive green spaces that are easily accessible. These features promote physical activity, reduce stress, and enhance overall well-being. A study by the Trust for Public Land (2020) found that neighborhoods of color have 50% less park space per capita than predominantly white neighborhoods. This deprives residents of safe areas to exercise, play, and connect with nature. Opposite to alluring, many Black neighborhoods are more likely to have cracked sidewalks, a lack of community centers, insufficient lighting, poorly marked streets, and potentially higher crime rates. All of which makes outdoor physical activity in one's own neighborhood less appealing and risky, rather than a truly viable option.

In clear contrast, predominantly white neighborhoods benefit from ongoing investments in infrastructure and amenities that promote health and safety. Meanwhile, the lack of public investment in Black community safety infrastructure further discourages outdoor activity, leading to an increase in the health disparities seen today. The lack of exercise-friendly environments in Black neighborhoods contributes to the higher rates of obesity, diabetes, and cardiovascular disease observed in these communities. Physical inactivity, combined with stress from unsafe conditions, accelerates the "weathering" effect described (in Chapter 4) by Dr. Arline Geronimus, wherein chronic exposure to stressors prematurely ages the body and increases vulnerability to disease. As Harriet Washington notes in *A Terrible Thing to Waste*, the geography of inequality is a geography of neglect, where environmental disrepair signals to Black communities that their health and well-being are of little concern to those in power. This lack of public investment in community safety infrastructure ultimately impairs the overall quality of life of its residents, as seen in the higher disease prevalence statistics.

Dismantling Public Safety Barriers

1. **Infrastructure Investment**: Allocate funding to improve sidewalks, lighting, and public transportation in historically neglected neighborhoods.

2. **Greenspace Development**: Increase access to parks and recreational facilities in communities of color.

3. **Community Policing Models**: Redefine law enforcement roles to prioritize building trust and collaboration with residents.

An example of efforts that exemplify barrier-breaking public safety initiatives includes:

MacGregor Park Revitalization in Houston's Third Ward: MacGregor Park, a 65-acre greenspace in Houston's historically Black Third Ward, is undergoing a $57.5 million transformation. The project focuses on ecological sustainability, native greenery, and improved safety features, including enhanced lighting and renovated sports facilities. This revitalization aims to provide a safe and inviting environment for community engagement and recreation.[171]

BARRIER NINE:
TRANSPORTATION AS AN OBSTACLE TO WELLNESS

Transportation is a fundamental social determinant of health, shaping access to employment, healthcare, education, and other essential resources. For African Americans, however, systemic racism embedded in transportation policies and infrastructure has created significant barriers. From the deliberate exclusion of public transit in predominantly white suburbs to inadequate safety measures at bus stops in Black neighborhoods, these inequities perpetuate cycles of disadvantage, poor health, and social exclusion.

The roots of transportation inequities lie in mid-20th-century urban renewal projects that prioritized highways over the well-being of Black communities. These projects often involved constructing highways directly through thriving Black neighborhoods, displacing residents and fracturing community cohesion. The construction of Interstate 40 in Nashville is a prime example, where a vibrant Black business district was decimated, leaving thousands of families uprooted and communities economically and socially isolated. The exclusion extended to public transit systems. In Atlanta, for instance, suburban counties like Cobb, Gwinnett, and Clayton actively resisted joining the Metropolitan Atlanta Rapid Transit Authority (MARTA), citing concerns about increased crime and "undesirable" populations—coded language for the growing number of Black residents. This resistance left many African Americans underserved by public transit, limiting their access to suburban job markets and further entrenching economic disparities. As transportation expert Robert Bullard points out, transportation inequities are not just about mobility; they are about access to opportunity. The exclusion of public transit from suburban areas is a deliberate strategy to segregate resources and limit economic mobility for African Americans.[172]

In many predominantly Black neighborhoods, public transit is often unreliable, infrequent, and geographically limited. According to a report by the Brookings Institution, African Americans are more likely to rely on public transportation than white Americans. Yet and still, they endure longer travel times and less consistent service.[173] This disparity reflects decades of disinvestment in transit infrastructure serving Black communities. This unreliability has a cascading effect on health and well-being. Without dependable transit, Black residents face barriers in accessing jobs, healthcare appointments, and education. A study published in JAMA Internal Medicine found that transportation barriers are a leading cause of missed medical appointments, which can delay critical diagnoses and treatments.[174] Transportation systems in Black neighborhoods often lack the necessary infrastructure for safety and comfort. Poorly marked bus stops, inadequate lighting, and a lack of benches and awnings leave residents vulnerable to accidents, weather exposure, and unsafe conditions. Women and children, in particular, face heightened safety risks when waiting for buses in dimly lit or isolated areas. Additionally, the absence of accessible transportation hubs in Black neighborhoods further limits mobility.

The health consequences of transportation inequities are severe and multifaceted. Unreliable transit systems and extended commutes disproportionately affect African Americans, many of whom work labor-intensive, low-wage jobs. These prolonged workdays, combined with the stress of navigating inadequate transit, increase the risk of hypertension, cardiovascular disease, and mental health challenges. Transit barriers contributing to missed or delayed medical appointments can result in a lack of treatment, follow-ups, or late-stage disease diagnoses, exacerbating health disparities. There is also a circular process of limited employment access, where individuals are unable to obtain or sustain employment in distant areas that may offer better wages and working conditions. This creates a perpetual cycle of barriers toward upward mobility, creating further mental and emotional distress that can lead to physical symptoms of limited financial resources and access to opportunities.

Solutions for Dismantling Transportation Barriers

1. **Public Transit Expansion**: Invest in expanding reliable and affordable public transit in underserved areas, including suburban job centers. Policies like tax incentives for transit companies and grants for urban transit development can help bridge gaps.

2. **Equity-Centered Policy Reform**: Advocate for transit policies that consider the needs of marginalized communities, such as fare reductions for low-income residents and prioritization of underserved routes.

3. **Safety and Accessibility Improvements**: Upgrade transit infrastructure with clear signage, adequate lighting, and benches or shelters at bus stops to improve safety and comfort.

An example of efforts that exemplify barrier-breaking transportation services initiatives includes:

Chicago's Far South Side Public Transit Expansion: In 2024, Chicago secured $1.9 billion in federal funding for a nearly $5.7

billion project to extend public transit to the city's far South Side. This initiative includes the addition of four new train stations, aiming to connect isolated, predominantly African American communities to the broader city infrastructure, thereby enhancing mobility and economic opportunities.[175]

BARRIER TEN:
IDENTITY AND STIGMA IN PUBLIC SPACES

Social identity, although not a typical SDH, plays a critical role in shaping an individual's self-esteem, sense of belonging, life satisfaction, and overall well-being, making it worth mentioning due to society's significant influence on it. For African Americans, the imposed identity of inferiority rooted in anti-Black racism has historically and contemporarily undermined this foundational aspect of health. This constructed narrative of inferiority is reinforced through systemic mechanisms, interpersonal interactions, and cultural representations, creating a feedback loop of oppression and negative self-perception. The cumulative effects of this devaluation profoundly influence not only self-perception provoked by societal treatment but also individual and collective health outcomes.

Historically, the media has played a significant role in shaping public perceptions of African Americans, often reinforcing stereotypes that perpetuate anti-Black racism. From the minstrel shows of the 19th century to early films like *The Birth of a Nation* (1915), which depicted Black men as dangerous and predatory, these portrayals were instrumental in reinforcing the justification for segregation, violence, and systemic discrimination. Such depictions created a cultural narrative that framed African Americans as inherently inferior, criminal, and unworthy of full citizenship. In the 20th century, the rise of television and film continued to perpetuate these harmful stereotypes. Black characters were often portrayed as maids, butlers, or criminals, roles that supported limited and/or demeaning societal views. For example, Mammy figures in films like *Gone with the Wind* (1939) reinforced the notion of Black women as servile and content in subjugation, while the caricature of the "lazy Black man" was proliferated in both visual and written media.

Contemporary media is not exempt from criticism. Studies have shown that news outlets are more likely to depict African Americans in stories about crime than whites. Statistics revealed the use of mugshots in 45% of cases that involved Black individuals accused of crimes, but only in 8% of cases involving white defendants. White victims were also nearly four times more likely to be presented in photos with friends and family than Black victims.[176] In addition, a study analyzing late-night news outlets in New York City found that the media reported on murder, theft, and assault cases involving Black suspects at rates exceeding their actual arrest statistics.[177] This overrepresentation in negative contexts fosters implicit biases among viewers, as evidenced by the results of the Harvard Implicit Association Test (IAT) on Race, which consistently demonstrates that a majority of participants, across racial groups, harbor an unconscious negative Black bias.

The true problem is that it does not stop at the level of influential societal biases; it grows into a more dangerous cycle of sustaining structural discrimination. For instance, research by the Pew Research Center found that African Americans are disproportionately targeted by police and receive harsher sentencing in the criminal justice system, outcomes often justified by the stereotype of inherent criminality. The negative social identity reinforced by media influences not only societal attitudes but also decision-making among those in positions of authority. In addition, when implicit biases are at play, little room is left for African Americans to receive the benefit of the doubt when discretionary decisions are involved. Implicit biases held by educators, healthcare providers, employers, and law enforcement officers can lead to unequal treatment of African Americans (as mentioned in previous sections). These biases not only limit opportunities but also reinforce the imposed social identity of inferiority, creating barriers to thriving and perpetuating a cycle of disadvantage.

The negative perceptions of African Americans are perpetuated through a circular process: biased media representations influence societal attitudes, which, in turn, inform institutional policies and interpersonal interactions. These policies and interactions then further reinforce the media's portrayal, creating a cycle that is difficult to escape. For African Americans, navigating a society that consistently devalues their identity is not only isolating but can ultimately be detrimental to health. Adding to the negative health impact of how biases show up in structural barriers, internalizing these negative messages can lead to diminished self-esteem, increased chronic stress, and a sense of hopelessness. The Doll Test conducted by Kenneth and Mamie Clark in the 1940s remains a powerful demonstration of how these messages affect young children. Black children in the study overwhelmingly preferred white dolls to Black dolls, associating whiteness with positive attributes and Blackness with negative ones. The most profound part of this test was the very telling look on their faces when they had to identify which one of the dolls looked most like them; it was a lightbulb moment as the children realized their connection to the doll they associated with all the negative characteristics. This early internalization of racial stigma has long-term implications for mental and emotional health because, if not disrupted with positive intentionality, these children can grow up into adults navigating these same internal battles.

Internalized beliefs often manifest in life and the body. Author Joy Degruy of *Post-Traumatic Slavery Syndrome* states that, "beliefs can so color our minds that we become paralyzed, unable to move beyond our fears and doubts, thus limiting our choices."[178] There is also a growing body of research quantifying how the internalization of negative stereotypes, the imposed narrative of Black inferiority, undermines healthy identity formation and is linked to adverse mental and even physical health outcomes. For instance, one longitudinal study of Black college students found that racial discrimination predicted increased anxiety symptoms, but only among those who already endorsed moderate to high levels of internalized negative stereotypes. In this study, the association between discrimination and later anxiety symptoms of distress was statistically significant at average and high levels of internalized negative stereotypes. In contrast, no significant relationship was observed for those with low levels of these internalized ideologies.[179] This pattern suggests that when Black individuals internalize messages of inferiority, experiences of discrimination are more likely to reinforce negative self-perceptions and trigger stress responses.

Complementing these findings, research by Mouzon and McLean (2016) compared mental health outcomes among African Americans, U.S.-born Caribbean Blacks, and foreign-born Caribbean Blacks. Their results showed that higher levels of internalized racism, reflecting the acceptance of culturally imposed notions of inferiority, were associated with significantly greater psychological distress and higher rates of depression among African Americans and US-born Caribbean Blacks relative to foreign-born Caribbean Blacks.[180] Together, these statistics support the idea that the imposed narrative of Black inferiority, when internalized, can compromise healthy identity formation and lead to measurable increases in mental health challenges. Black immigrants being introduced to the lived Black experience of being swarmed with negative stereotypes from multiple outlets reasonably creates this internalization if Black people are not receiving counter messages of positivity at an equal or greater rate than negative messages. Over time, internalized oppression may also contribute to chronic physiological stress (for example, through higher allostatic load), thereby linking these psychological processes with adverse physical health outcomes.

Negative stereotypes are more than a notion. When internalized, it sows seeds of limitation around self-perception and ambitions that blossom into self-doubt. This can influence the trajectory of one's entire life. It can deter African Americans from seeking advancement opportunities due to fear of rejection or failure, which are tied to societal biases. A study examining the influence of internalized racism on African American adults' career aspirations found a negative correlation between internalized negative stereotypes and career goals. Participants who internalized these stereotypes tended to set lower career aspirations, limiting their professional growth and opportunities.[181] Research indicates that internalized racism contributes to a fear of failure among African Americans, particularly in educational settings. This fear can discourage individuals from applying to colleges or pursuing higher education due to concerns about potential rejection or academic difficulties. Such apprehensions are often reinforced by societal messages questioning their intellectual capabilities. The internalization of negative stereotypes is associated with increased psychological distress, including anxiety and depression, which can further erode self-esteem and reinforce self-doubt, creating a cycle that hinders both personal and professional development.

Systemic discrimination and societal expectations clearly play a significant role in perpetuating these challenges of internalized racism. The U.S. workforce system, for instance, has been reported to restrict opportunities for Black Americans through discriminatory practices, often channeling them into low-wage jobs with limited prospects for advancement in responsibilities or pay. This systemic bias can reinforce negative self-perceptions and potentially deter individuals from pursuing higher ambitions. Attempting to thrive past these hurdles lends credence to understanding why representation matters in all industries and fields of study. Cultural representation can help foster an internal sense of hope and possibility in future generations to aspire to careers with a more compelling grip beyond societal-imposed limitations.

As indicated, the health consequences of internalized racism are profound. In America, being constantly bombarded with negative stereotypes and discrimination is almost inescapable for many Blacks, thereby contributing to a reduction in overall life satisfaction and fostering feelings of hopelessness and despair. Chronic stress resulting from a devalued social identity triggers prolonged activation of the body's stress response, leading to systemic inflammation, hypertension, and increased risk of cardiovascular disease. Additionally, feelings of inferiority can lead to maladaptive coping mechanisms, such as substance abuse, overeating, or social withdrawal, further exacerbating health disparities. A sense of powerlessness and lack of agency, cultivated by centuries of systemic oppression, contributes to a cycle of survival rather than thriving. In a society where structural barriers persist, the mental toll of fighting against these odds daily creates a significant added burden on health and well-being that can impact generations.

Solutions for Empowering Positive Social Identity

1. **Culturally Responsive Education**: Integrating Black history and achievements into school curricula to foster pride and counteract negative stereotypes.

2. **Media Representation**: Expanding the portrayal of Black individuals to reflect diverse, empowered, and authentic identities that showcase their resilience, achievements, and humanity.

3. **Mental Health Interventions**: Providing accessible, culturally competent mental health resources to help individuals process and resist internalized racism.

An example of efforts that exemplify barrier-breaking in social identity includes:

New York City's Black Studies Curriculum Expansion: In August 2024, New York City public schools introduced a comprehensive Black Studies Curriculum aimed at integrating Black history and achievements across subjects like arts, English, and history. This initiative seeks to deepen students' understanding of Black heritage and foster pride within the community.[182]

PART TWO CONCLUSION

The social determinants of health are not passive background factors; they are active, daily barriers that shape every aspect of life for

African Americans. Housing instability, limited access to quality education, chronic underemployment, food deserts, and unequal access to health services are not isolated issues. Instead, they work in tandem, forming an interconnected web of obstacles that undermine well-being at every stage of life. When compounded with environmental hazards, unsafe neighborhoods, unreliable transportation, and the added burden of navigating public spaces while carrying a marginalized social identity, the cumulative impact is devastating. These are not occasional stressors. They are constant, inescapable conditions that wear down the body, mind, and spirit, driving the high rates of chronic illness we see today in Black communities.

The reality is undeniable: if an individual is not overwhelmed by the health consequences of one barrier, another barrier is often waiting just a few feet away to stifle progress towards thriving in life. The relentless nature of these overlapping inequities limits not only individual potential but also the collective advancement of entire communities. Over time, this continuous strain becomes health-limiting, embedding itself into the daily experience of Black life. It is no wonder that disease prevalence, early mortality, and chronic health conditions remain disproportionately high. Living under the weight of structural inequities, without reprieve, creates an environment where the pursuit of health becomes an uphill battle, fought on multiple fronts, throughout the day, every day.

For guided discussion questions and activities, visit:
https://wellnessedu.blackcellconsulting.com
to access your FREE REFLECTION GUIDE.

PART III:
THE BIOLOGY OF OPPRESSION

Black Wellness Barriers

While the physical and psychological dehumanization of slavery laid the foundation for generational trauma, the legacy of these historical abuses lives on—not only in cultural memory but within the bodies of African Americans today. Part III of this book explores how centuries of oppression have translated into tangible, measurable health consequences, as the relentless pressures of racial discrimination, systemic violence, and economic exclusion keep Black communities trapped in chronic states of survival.

This phenomenon isn't merely abstract. In a Pew Research Center study, nearly half of Black adults reported adverse health outcomes directly linked to experiences of discrimination. One participant reflected, "I've had moments at work where a comment or look reminded me exactly how I was perceived, and suddenly my heart was racing. I felt my whole body tense up. I carried that feeling home. It lingered long after the moment passed."

Oppressive conditions in America have not only shaped lived experiences—they have altered physiological processes, creating a persistent cycle of stress-related disease and early mortality. This section examines how the biology of stress, triggered by ongoing racial inequities, drives higher rates of hypertension, cardiovascular disease, diabetes, and other chronic illnesses that disproportionately affect African Americans.

Yet the impact of oppression extends beyond immediate stress responses. Emerging research in the field of epigenetics reveals that the trauma endured by oppressed people has been passed down across generations, leaving biological imprints that continue to affect health today. Through cross-cultural comparisons—such as studies of Holocaust survivors and the Dutch Hunger Winter—as well as findings from the New York African Burial Ground, we begin to understand how historical trauma leaves its mark on DNA, influencing disease risk decades or even centuries later.

In addition, the developmental origins of the health and disease framework highlight how early-life exposures—whether in the womb or during childhood—shape long-term health outcomes. From birth, many African Americans are disproportionately burdened by the compounded weight of historical and contemporary trauma. Together, these chapters illuminate how deeply the past is woven into the present, not only socially and psychologically, but also within the very physiology of Black bodies in America.

CHAPTER 4:
UNDER PRESSURE: CHRONIC STRESS AND THE LIVED BLACK EXPERIENCE

> "Maybe you've known what it is to leave your body to survive. And maybe when the threat has subsided, you've been unable to find your way back. This racist, capitalist, ableist world does not want to keep you whole. It can only stand to benefit from bodies emptied of their protectors. But hear this: If you aren't in your body, someone else is. You will too soon find that the many tyrants of the world have taken the helm in your absence. For this reason, our liberation practice must be tied to a reclamation of the physical self—to an embodied homecoming. Just as our spiritualities draw us into our interior worlds, they should also be a map back home to our bodies, a mirror held to our very faces."
> - Cole Arthur Riley, *Black Liturgies*

The human body is naturally designed to self-protect, self-repair, and self-preserve because it is hard-wired for survival. One of the most fundamental mechanisms for this self-preservation is the stress response—a biological cascade triggered when the brain perceives a threat, real or imagined. This response activates the hypothalamic-pituitary-adrenal (HPA) axis, flooding the body with hormones like cortisol and adrenaline to prepare for immediate action. Heart rate increases, blood pressure rises, and glucose is released into the bloodstream—all in service of survival.

PART III: THE BIOLOGY OF OPPRESSION

In acute situations, this physiological alarm system is lifesaving. But when continually activated by non-life-threatening, chronic stressors—like racism, microaggressions, and economic instability—the very mechanism meant to protect the body begins to wear it down. The stress response was designed to be brief and infrequent, but for many African Americans, it becomes a constant state of engagement.

Part III of this book explores how this biological reality intersects with systemic inequity. The daily lived experiences of Black Americans often leave no room for sustained disengagement of the stress response. Chronic stress becomes normalized. Pew focus group participant noted, "It wasn't until my doctor pointed out that my blood pressure spikes after certain work meetings that I realized my body was literally reacting like I was in physical danger. It's a survival response, but I didn't see it clearly until I saw it as numbers on a page."

Another woman, quoted in a BuzzFeed collection on health disparities among Black women, described the toll of cumulative emotional labor: "I was exhausted, constantly. Every meeting, every interaction, felt loaded with tension. Doctors said my fatigue was psychological, but eventually, tests showed the physical toll—high blood pressure, inflammation markers off the charts. My body was trying to tell a story, but no one was listening." These stories are not isolated. Research shows that racism-induced stress contributes to physiological changes that disproportionately affect African Americans. Chronic stress is more than psychological—it disrupts immune function, accelerates aging, and drives chronic inflammation, which in turn increases vulnerability to hypertension, cardiovascular disease, diabetes, and more.

Contemporary stressors no longer require us to flee from predators, but the body still reacts as if it must. Being called a racial slur, navigating tokenism in the workplace, or reliving a traumatic interaction all activate the same emergency systems. Over time, these repeated activations prevent the body from returning to a state of balance—homeostasis—turning a protective response into a source of harm.

To be Black in America is, for many, to adapt to chronic stress as a way of life. But biology cannot normalize what is inherently abnormal. The body keeps the score; over time, the cost becomes visible in bloodwork, diagnoses, and mortality rates.

The Inflammation Connection: How Chronic Stress Wreaks Biological Havoc

Chronic stress goes beyond emotional discomfort—it physically alters our bodies. It disrupts immune function, accelerates aging, and triggers chronic inflammation, often called "silent inflammation." This type of inflammation quietly fuels conditions such as heart disease, diabetes, obesity, autoimmune diseases, and neurological disorders.[183] Research consistently shows that African Americans have higher baseline levels of inflammation markers—like C-reactive protein (CRP) and interleukin-6 (IL-6)—indicating a constantly activated immune system, which contributes significantly to disease and premature death.[184]

Continuous exposure to stressors, such as racial discrimination, economic hardship, or traumatic life experiences, keeps the body's stress response permanently activated, amplifying inflammation and increasing disease risk. According to researcher David R. Williams, racial discrimination alone significantly raised inflammatory markers like CRP and fibrinogen, even after controlling for other lifestyle factors.[185]

Cortisol usually helps regulate inflammation by calming the immune response. However, prolonged stress disrupts cortisol regulation, causing the immune system to become either overly active or insufficiently responsive, leading to chronic inflammation.[186] African Americans, disproportionately exposed to structural oppression and chronic stress, frequently experience disrupted cortisol rhythms, placing them at higher risk for inflammatory diseases such as hypertension, diabetes, and cardiovascular conditions. Over time, this chronic inflammation accelerates biological aging and increases vulnerability to disease.

Arline Geronimus, who coined the term "weathering," highlights how constant stress gradually erodes health over a lifetime, disproportionately affecting African Americans regardless of socioeconomic status.[187] Chronic stress has also been shown to shorten telomeres—the protective caps at the ends of chromosomes—which leads to premature aging and heightened disease vulnerability, disproportionately impacting African Americans compared to other groups.[188] These physical outcomes are not happening in a vacuum; they are the biological consequences of living within systems that maintain inequality. Part II of this book explored the societal structures—housing, education, food access, health care, and more—that fuel the chronic stress response at every turn.

This link between chronic stress, inflammation, and adverse health outcomes is vividly illustrated in Cheryl L. Woods-Giscombé's qualitative research exploring the "Superwoman Schema" among African American women. Her study captures how internalizing stress and embodying resilience as an expected social role can exact a profound physical toll. One participant reflected:

> "My Nana was the strongest person I knew. She never showed her pain—never cried, never complained. She silently endured diabetes, obesity, breast cancer, and even a double mastectomy. Later, I learned she'd experienced a nervous breakdown as a younger woman. After she passed, I realized how much suffering she might have avoided if she'd felt safe enough to express her pain openly. It made me question, was that strength really strength if it broke her down physically?"[189]

This story demonstrates powerfully how the silent burden of chronic stress not only shapes personal experiences but leaves tangible biological marks that drive illness and shorten life.

Stroke, Heart Disease, and the Weight of Survival

The link between psychosocial stress and hypertension is well-documented in medical literature. For African Americans, the stress of navigating racist social structures and their associated factors leads to a sustained "fight-or-flight" physiological state.[190] This constant activation of the sympathetic nervous system can result in: Repeated surges in cortisol and adrenaline, increased vascular resistance leading to chronic hypertension, and accelerated arterial calcification that will contribute to early cardiovascular aging. These are major contributing factors to heart disease risk, as indicated in a research study published in NEJM that highlights that African Americans are at a higher risk of developing heart failure at a younger age.[191] Such a deadly cycle of disease may be associated with early-onset conditions like hypertension and obesity, both of which can be triggered by stress.

According to the CDC 2017 Vital Signs, African Americans ages 35-64 are 50% more likely to have high blood pressure than their white counterparts. The alarming disparities become more stark considering that hypertension increases the risk of strokes. Strokes happen when the arterial blood flow, which carries oxygen and nutrients, is blocked in a part of the brain. Statistics show that Blacks ages 45-54 have a mortality rate 3 times that of their white counterparts.[192] Research has also shown that racial discrimination directly contributes to higher blood pressure levels in African Americans. In a Jackson Heart study, findings indicate that stress from lifetime discrimination is associated with an increased risk of hypertension among African Americans.[193] The stress response triggered by repeated oppressive encounters leads to chronic activation and dysregulation of the hypothalamic-pituitary-adrenal (HPA) axis, increasing blood pressure that can damage arteries and blood vessels over time.

Compounding the physiology of stress with psychosocial environmental factors culminates in the impact of John Henryism. This concept, introduced by Dr. Sherman James, describes a high-effort

PART III: THE BIOLOGY OF OPPRESSION

coping strategy commonly seen among African Americans who continuously exert intense mental and physical energy to overcome systemic racism, economic hardship, and social exclusion.[194] Rooted in the folklore of the steel-driving man John Henry, this coping style reflects a cultural expectation of resilience and relentless hard work in the face of oppressive conditions. However, the prolonged exertion required to "push through" structural barriers, often without adequate rest, resources, or support, takes a severe toll on the body. Arline Geronimus points out many studies indicating that "Black working class, being high in John Henryism, predicts higher mean blood pressure, obesity, and other risk factors for cardiovascular disease and cancer."[195] Thus, for many African Americans, the combination of external racism-induced stress and internalized high-effort coping creates a double burden that significantly increases health risks, further embedding racial health disparities within the lived Black experience.

An example of John Henryism is seen in Christian, a sophomore at Emory University at the time of the interview, as he reflects on the racialized aspects of his lived experience as a Black male on campus. He speaks very candidly about the compounded stressors of navigating both the academic rigor and daily Black life that he admits is a fatiguing process, particularly when, "You have to sit there and explain stuff to people, and it's tiring because you end up being the person who has to come to the defense of Blackness all the time even if you don't want to."[196] Christian is well aware of the potential negative impact racial biases and judgments from his professors and colleagues can have on the Black community, especially if those ignorant perspectives are left unchallenged. Outspoken Black voices are commonly not welcomed in white-dominant spaces, yet that does not curtail the role Christian chooses to play in resisting the spread of more racially cited ignorance when encountered.

There is a physical tax the body can end up paying as these cumulative stressors add up over time. On a cellular level, his body manages behind the scenes how his presence on campus leaves him vulnerable to daily forms of disrespect on a macro and micro level of aggression. Christian regularly experiences other students treating him like he is inferior. His maladaptation to these experiences leaves him feeling like making any kind of mistake is not an option or that anger is an emotion he has to repress because expressing it is too consequential. As a protective shield from preconceived assumptions of not belonging on campus, Christian states, "Feel the need to literally wear Emory gear everywhere he goes so that people don't think he is just some random person, and I hate doing it."[197] Sometimes his labeled clothing is not enough when the blackness of his skin dominates their perception of him as a threat. Particularly in the case of a female Indian student who ran across the street late one night once she spotted Christian, dressed in Emory-branded clothing from head to toe, walking across campus.

Blood Sugar and Body Size: Racialized Metabolism

The cumulative effects of chronic stress exposure have profound consequences on metabolic health, especially for the African American population that experiences higher rates of obesity, type 2 diabetes, and metabolic syndrome, all of which are significantly influenced by stress-related hormonal imbalances and systemic inflammation.[198] Chronic stress increases cortisol production, which promotes fat storage, particularly in the abdominal region, leading to higher obesity rates and insulin resistance. According to the Nutrition Examination Survey (NHANES) 2017-2018 study, the prevalence of obesity was highest (56.9%) among African American women 20 years of age and older.[199] Carrying additional adipose tissue (fat) feeds into the cycle of persistent inflammation that impairs glucose metabolism, fosters insulin resistance, and eventually leads to type 2 diabetes and potential beta cell failure. The progressive health impact of those extra pounds translates into data from the American Diabetes Association, which shows that African Americans are almost twice as likely to develop diabetes compared to their white counterparts.[200] Further diabetes statistics reveal that in

2020, Black patients were admitted to the hospital for uncontrolled diabetes at nearly four times the rate as whites, and in 2021, they were 40% more likely to die from diabetes.[201]

Socioeconomic instability and its associated systemic stressors, which also include food insecurity and environmental toxins, equate to a compounded risk that places African Americans in an environment that exacerbates poor metabolic health outcomes. There are many paths down the deadly road of chronic stress, triggering excessive cortisol production that heightens the risk for metabolic syndrome and cardiovascular disease. When the body is flooded with cortisol from chronic stress, it increases appetite not just for anything but cravings specifically for high-fat and/or high-sugar foods that help to diminish the emotions associated with the stress response. Therefore, the body experiences the physiological impact of excessive fats and sugars to process while already being flooded with excess, underutilized glucose from the stress response. This vicious cycle tips the scales toward packing on the pounds and other increased metabolic risks. It doesn't stop there; the cumulative impact of these stress-induced inflammatory pathways also contributes to a feedback circuit of physiological dysregulation stimulated from multiple angles that reinforces the disparities in metabolic health. What further deepens the racial gap in chronic disease prevalence and mortality is the higher exposure to economic stressors, racial discrimination, and limited healthcare access. These structural barriers experienced as stressors make it more challenging for African Americans to manage these conditions effectively, resulting in higher rates of complications such as kidney disease, amputations, and neuropathy.[202]

Immunity Compromised: How Racism Weakens the Body's Defenses

Chronic stress burdens the cardiovascular system and metabolic pathways and fundamentally weakens the immune system, increasing susceptibility to infections, autoimmune disorders, and chronic inflammation. For African Americans, whose lives are often shaped by persistent social and structural inequitable barriers, the impact of stress on immune function is especially concerning. The body's ability to defend itself against pathogens, repair cellular damage, and maintain long-term health is significantly compromised when in a constant state of fight or flight.

African Americans have been found to have higher allostatic loads, meaning greater physiological wear and tear due to prolonged exposure to stress hormones like cortisol and adrenaline.[203] The prolonged secretion of cortisol, the body's primary stress hormone, lowers the effectiveness of white blood cells (lymphocytes) in fighting infections.[204] Chronic stress can also cause immune cell aging, known as immunosenescence, which reduces the body's ability to respond to new infections and exacerbates existing vulnerabilities. The COVID-19 pandemic blatantly illuminated longstanding racial health disparities in the United States. Black Americans faced disproportionately high rates of infection and mortality, outcomes rooted not only in pre-existing health conditions but also in deeply entrenched systemic inequities. While much of the nation had the privilege of staying at home to reduce their exposure and protect others, many Black Americans, particularly those employed in essential service roles, did not have that option. For them, continuing to work in public-facing jobs was not a choice but a financial necessity driven by economic survival.

This economic vulnerability, coupled with chronic stress, systemic inflammation, and overrepresentation in high-risk occupations, significantly increased exposure to the virus. Limited access to quality healthcare further compounded these risks. The combined burden of physical exposure and social stressors magnified the pandemic's impact on Black communities, revealing how the structure of American labor and health systems leaves the most vulnerable with the least protection in times of crisis.

From Cancer to Conception: The Hidden Reach of Chronic Stress

The role of chronic stress in cancer risk is often overlooked. Yet, emerging research suggests that stress plays a significant role in cancer initiation, progression, and mortality rates, particularly for African Americans. Chronic psychological and physiological stress can promote cancer development by suppressing immune function, increasing systemic inflammation, and creating an environment conducive to tumor growth.[205] African Americans experience higher rates of many cancers and worse survival outcomes compared to their white counterparts. According to the American Cancer Society, "Black men have a 67% higher prostate cancer incidence rate compared to white men and are more than twice as likely to die from the disease."[206] Meanwhile, the same source reveals that, although Black women have 5% lower rates of being diagnosed with breast cancer, they are 38% more likely to die from it compared to white women. This racial disparity is partially attributable to differences in healthcare access and socioeconomic factors. Still, chronic stress has emerged as a critical, yet underrecognized, contributor to cancer risk in this population.[207]

When the body is subjected to long-term stress, the hypothalamic-pituitary-adrenal (HPA) axis becomes dysregulated, producing excessive cortisol and norepinephrine. These stress hormones promote tumor cell survival, inhibit apoptosis (programmed cell death), and stimulate the formation of new blood vessels that feed tumors.[208] African Americans face greater exposure to socioeconomic and racial stressors, which are often embedded in the daily structures of life. This persistent stress burden is reflected biologically, with studies showing that African Americans tend to have higher baseline levels of cortisol, the body's primary stress hormone. Elevated stress sets off a cascade of health risks, including heightened vulnerability to cancer, and chronic cortisol over time increases the risk of stress-induced cellular damage, compromising the body's resilience to disease.[209] The relentless strain of navigating systemic racism, often referred to as racial stress, contributes to premature cellular aging. One clear marker is the shortening of telomeres—protective caps at the ends of chromosomes that naturally erode with age. According to Geronimus, marginalized populations contend with increased exposure to multi-tiered environmental stressors, which speeds up telomere shortening, thereby making groups like African Americans more susceptible to quicker biological aging.[210] This erosion sets off a cascade of health risks, including heightened vulnerability to cancer and other previously mentioned chronic diseases. The cumulative nature of these stressors doesn't just affect isolated systems; it produces widespread physiological impact. In this way, every layer of exposure is interconnected, highlighting the multi-layered pathway between structural racism and health disparities.

Chronic stress also correlates with systemic inflammation, a well-documented driver of cancer progression. As previously mentioned, African Americans exhibit higher levels of inflammatory markers such as interleukin-6 (IL-6) and C-reactive protein (CRP), which are associated with both chronic stress exposure and tumor growth.[211] Given that African Americans experience greater exposure to environmental toxins, food insecurity, and the neglect of medical institutions, the combined effects of chronic inflammation and stress-induced immune dysfunction make them more vulnerable to both developing and dying from aggressive cancers. The desolate reality is that even when diagnosed, Black cancer patients often face worse treatment outcomes due to systemic barriers to healthcare access. Black patients facing socioeconomic barriers may be financially ineligible for advanced care treatments, such as immunotherapy, when recipients are using Medicare versus private insurance to pay for healthcare expenses.[212] Other healthcare limitations, including the form of implicit bias among healthcare providers, economic inequality, and historical medical mistrust, can all contribute to delayed diagnoses and lower treatment adherence, all providing a feedback loop into the cycle of stress.

Reproductive Health

Reproductive health is another crucial area of health that is often overlooked regarding how chronic stress impacts Black women. For centuries, Black women in America have faced a unique and dispro-

PART III: THE BIOLOGY OF OPPRESSION

portionate burden when it comes to maternal health. Their bodies have been subjected to systemic violence, chronic stress, environmental hazards, medical neglect, and economic deprivation, all of which have left an imprint on their reproductive health and that of their descendants. The maternal health crisis facing Black women today is not a coincidence; it is a direct consequence of historical oppression, ongoing structural racism, and intergenerational stress transmission. The biological consequences of stress, particularly the overproduction of cortisol and inflammatory markers, are increasingly recognized as major contributors to reproductive disorders, pregnancy complications, and infant mortality.

Fertility

Despite the common misconception that Black women are naturally hyper-fertile, research indicates that infertility rates are higher among African American women compared to their white counterparts.[213] Chronic stress triggers the hypothalamic-pituitary-adrenal (HPA) axis, producing excess cortisol. Prolonged cortisol exposure can disrupt ovulation, lower progesterone levels, and increase the risk of pregnancy loss.[214] There are also stress-related chronic inflammation, metabolic disorders, and hormonal imbalances, such as polycystic ovary syndrome (PCOS), which disproportionately affects Black women and serves as a major contributor to infertility. Exposure to environmental toxins due to ecological racism (e.g., air pollution, endocrine disruptors in hair and beauty products) has also been linked to disrupted menstrual cycles, higher rates of fibroids, and reduced fertility. The stress associated with fertility leaves African American women hurdling further disadvantages that include financing, use of, and success of assisted reproductive technology like In Vitro Fertilization (IVF), medical distrust, and limited healthcare access in their pursuits to motherhood.

Maternal Health & Birth Outcomes

There is a present-day maternal health crisis among Black women that continues to be both driven by and further contributing to healthcare disparities. Among those are racial stressors that include medical racism, workplace discrimination, and financial instability, which amplify these reproductive health risks for Black women, putting them among the highest in the industrialized world for maternal mortality. According to the CDC, African American women are three times more likely to die from pregnancy-related complications than white women, regardless of education or income.[215] One of the leading complications is Preeclampsia (characterized by dangerously high blood pressure spikes typically after 20 weeks of pregnancy), which can be triggered by chronic stressors. Black women are not only 60% more likely to develop preeclampsia and twice as likely to suffer severe complications from the condition compared to white women, but sadly, this gestational condition increases their risk of heart failure later in life.[216] Compounded with the chronic stress of being a Black woman, other pre-existing conditions such as chronic hypertension and obesity can elevate preeclampsia prevalence as well. The crisis is so pervasive that numerous organizations try but struggle to keep up with the need to provide support, life-saving advocacy, and sadly, resources on grief for Black mothers, and the surviving family members of both moms and babies that are part of the astounding statistics on inequity. An article from *The Root* describes one such effort: "Erica McAfee was searching for support after experiencing stillbirth and miscarriage. So she started Sisters in Loss, an organization that supports women dealing with pregnancy or infant loss and infertility. They provide educational and doula services in pregnancy, birth, and postpartum bereavement, as well as grief support so that women can find peace after loss."[217]

Pre-Term and Low Birth Weight Newborns

Birth weight and preterm births serve as critical indicators of lifelong health outcomes and disproportionately affect African American births at higher rates. Current studies reveal their preterm births at 14.6% and low birth weight at 13%, ranking Blacks at the highest among other racial and ethnic groups.[218] African Americans have consistently faced disproportionately higher rates of low birth weight (defined as less than 2,500 grams /or 5.5 lbs.) and preterm births (delivery before 37 weeks of gestation), both of which significantly increase the risk of chronic health conditions and mortality throughout the human lifespan. The physiological stress endured by Black mothers, compounded by systemic and interpersonal racism, has been shown to directly impact these birth outcomes, creating a ripple effect that extends into adulthood. Low birth weight and preterm births are associated with a range of adverse health outcomes, including higher risks of hypertension, insulin resistance, diabetes, cardiovascular disease (CVD), and neurodevelopmental disorders in the offspring. Infants born prematurely often have underdeveloped organs, particularly the lungs, heart, and brain, which can lead to respiratory issues, developmental delays, and learning disabilities. These early vulnerabilities can exacerbate disparities in educational attainment, employment opportunities, and overall quality of life, further entrenching systemic inequities.

A study conducted by the CDC found that Black women experience preterm births at a rate nearly 50% higher than white women. Alarmingly, this disparity persists even when accounting for socioeconomic factors. For example, college-educated Black women are nearly twice as likely to have low-birth-weight babies compared to their college-educated white counterparts. Unfortunately, the alarming differences don't stop there; CDC statistics also revealed that even when compared to white women without high school diplomas, Black women with college degrees still had worse low birth weight outcomes.[219] These findings underscore the role of systemic racism and chronic stress as primary drivers of adverse birth outcomes, rather than socioeconomic status alone. Geronimus' Weathering Hypothesis suggests that Black women's bodies age faster due to prolonged stress, leading to complications during pregnancy that mirror those of much older white women.[220] This premature aging further complicates an already compromised internal cellular environment and external lived environment for the African American female to reproduce optimally.

When the Mind Carries the Burden

The body is not the only aspect of one's well-being affected by stress. Chronic stress profoundly impacts the brain's ability to process emotions, regulate behavior, and make decisions, with long-term consequences for cognitive function. From historical trauma to contemporary microaggressions, the effects of stress are compounded across generations, creating profound implications for cognitive function, emotional resilience, and overall mental well-being. The physiological response to stress, particularly cortisol dysregulation, neuroinflammation, and impaired executive function, places individuals at increased risk for anxiety, depression, cognitive decline, and trauma-related disorders.

Scientific data shows that excessive cortisol can damage neural structures, with one of the most vulnerable areas being the hippocampus, a region in the brain crucial for memory formation, learning, and adaptive thinking.[221] Prolonged exposure to stress-related neurotoxicity impairs an individual's ability to recall information, concentrate, and effectively problem-solve, which can make it challenging to escape harmful situations or strategize for a better future. Studies suggest that chronic stress and systemic inflammation accelerate cognitive decline, further widening racial disparities in neurodegenerative diseases.[222] Evidence of these disparities is seen in recent studies demonstrating that African Americans are twice as likely to develop Alzheimer's disease and other forms of dementia compared to white Americans, even when controlling for genetic factors.[223]

Historically, for enslaved Africans, this neurological disruption compounded their inability to resist or escape their conditions. This state of chronic cognitive overload likely contributed to learned helplessness, a psychological state in which individuals, after repeated exposure to uncontrollable stressors, begin to perceive resistance as futile and resign themselves to their conditions. Contemporarily, the Black population continues to navigate the treacherous terrain of overt discrimination, microaggressions, and other structural inequi-

PART III: THE BIOLOGY OF OPPRESSION

ties in their personal experience. Leading to data revealing that Black adults exposed to chronic stress had significantly lower cognitive function compared to their white counterparts, even when adjusting for education and socioeconomic status.[224] All this, combined with limited access to mental health resources, exacerbates the mental health crisis seen among African Americans.

Another area of the brain of significant concern is the amygdala, which regulates fear, anxiety, and emotional processing and becomes hyperactive in individuals who experience chronic stress and trauma. The constant state of hypervigilance and fear, necessary for survival in an environment where brutal punishment was an ever-present threat, made it difficult for enslaved Blacks to focus on anything beyond immediate self-preservation. This heightened vigilance kept them in what researchers Williams and Mohammad call "prolonged physiological activation," which can contribute to difficulty managing decompressing from high emotional responses to the perceived threat of discriminatory stressors.[225] The persistent fear can be attributed to historical trauma, racial profiling, police violence, and workplace discrimination, to name a few. All of which contributes to chronic hypervigilance that can eventually exhaust the nervous system and deplete mental resilience.

Beyond cognitive impairments, enslavement also took an immense toll on emotional regulation, reinforcing generational patterns of psychological distress that persist in Black communities today. Enslaved people were routinely forced to suppress their natural emotional responses to oppression; any defiance, expressed through anger, grief, or even an assertion of dignity, could result in violent retaliation. This emotional suppression was a survival mechanism, but it came at a devastating cost. Studies indicate that bottling up emotions leads to heightened physiological stress responses.[226] Suppressing feelings in the moment as a perpetual survival strategy can lead to increased blood pressure, chronic anxiety, and depressive symptoms. Enslaved individuals, unable to fully process their grief over lost loved ones, stolen autonomy, and daily dehumanization, likely experienced deep psychological distress, compounded by the lack of safe spaces to express or heal from their suffering. These conditions fostered chronic emotional dysregulation, a state that modern research has linked to the intergenerational transmission of trauma, particularly in populations that have endured systemic oppression (to be discussed in Chapter 5).

This historical burden of psychological distress compounds with present-day oppressive conditions that offer no reprieve for the Black population. There is a self-internalized pressure for Black women and men to "stay strong," resisting the urge to be too expressive, too emotional, or too loud, all of which get a negative label of "angry Black woman" or "aggressive Black man" attached to it. Silence can become self-sacrificing to their health and well-being in the struggle towards equity in the workplace, communities, or society-at-large. A perpetual fight to be seen, heard, and respected is not sustainable by any means, as detailed by Mary Frances Winters in her book *Black Fatigue: How Racism Erodes the Mind, Body, and Spirit.*[227] Not only is dodging career-destroying labels downright fatiguing, but it can also lead to mental and emotional exhaustion. Navigating this sense of elevated depletion only escalates when mental health conditions among African Americans, who statistically are underdiagnosed and/or undertreated due to associated social stigmas, healthcare access, and access to racially concordant or culturally competent mental health providers.

Lastly, the psychological impact of racial trauma is profound, persistent, and often underrecognized in mainstream mental health spaces. While Post-Traumatic Stress Disorder (PTSD) is typically associated with acute, life-threatening experiences such as military combat or physical assault, the trauma experienced by African Americans is both historical and ongoing, with no definitive endpoint in sight. Racial trauma, a form of PTSD caused by prolonged exposure to racism, discrimination, and systemic oppression, has been found to produce many of the same psychological and physiological symptoms as traditional PTSD Symptoms include: hypervigilance, anxiety, depression, and emotional dysregulation. However, what distinguishes racial trauma from other forms of PTSD is that it is transgenerational, passed down through family and community narratives, cultural memory, and lived experiences, reinforcing the psychological burden of navigating a world structured by anti-Black racism. Joy DeGruy's *Post-Traumatic Slave Syndrome* (PTSS) framework expands upon this idea, arguing that the multi-century trauma of enslavement, followed by the brutality of segregation and continued structural racism, has created a collective and enduring psychological wound within the African American community.[228] This unresolved trauma manifests in self-destructive behaviors, internalized oppression, and a deeply ingrained mistrust of institutions, particularly those historically complicit in Black suffering.

One of the most damaging aspects of PTSS is the internalization of inferiority, which is directly tied to historical trauma. Through epigenetic changes and social conditioning, oppressive stressors have shaped emotional and cognitive health outcomes in African Americans today. Centuries of racist policies, violent oppression, and cultural erasure have conditioned many African Americans to adopt the very narratives designed to dehumanize them subconsciously. This internalized oppression can present itself as self-doubt, low self-worth, and the belief that success is unattainable. This erosion of confidence not only diminishes self-esteem, but it also discourages pursuits of career and educational advancements that can reinforce the cycle of racial disadvantage. Psychological studies have shown that chronic exposure to racial discrimination leads to heightened stress responses, wearing down mental resilience over time, and contributing to a sense of learned helplessness.[229] Furthermore, these negative self-perceptions are often reinforced by structural barriers such as educational inequities, employment discrimination, and biased policing, creating a circular relationship in which African Americans struggle to overcome both external oppression and the internalized belief of being inherently less capable.

Searching for Reprieve

As pointed out throughout this chapter, "Racism is one of the most prominent stressors in African Americans' everyday lives and leads to a host of detrimental outcomes. African Americans who report experiencing racial discrimination have reported low levels of well-being, greater anger expression, and higher depressive symptoms." Therefore, learning how to cope with and mitigate these stressors is vital. Out of an extensive range of strategies that Black people use to respond to the various forms of racism, research shows that coping strategies are most widely used, regardless of gender, including emotional regulation, religion, social support, and problem-focused management. More about mitigation strategies will be discussed in Chapter 7.

When confronted with persistent racial stressors, whether through microaggressions, systemic inequities, or the internal weight of generational trauma, many African Americans find themselves turning to coping behaviors that, while offering short-term relief, can ultimately contribute to long-term harm. Chronic exposure to racism has been linked to increased use of substances like tobacco, alcohol, and high-fat or high-sugar comfort foods as a means of numbing or managing emotional pain. These behaviors, while socially normalized in some contexts, are often responses to a more profound sense of powerlessness, exhaustion, or unresolved grief. Studies show that emotional eating, substance use, and even chronic sleep disruption are more prevalent in populations facing structural oppression, serving as quiet but significant indicators of distress masked as everyday habits.[230]

Moreover, from a psychological perspecitve, the emotional toll of racial stress often leads to coping strategies like suppression, avoidance, and rumination. For example, some individuals may choose not to speak up in the face of discrimination to maintain employment, safety, or social peace—an act of expressive suppression that can lead to internalized stress, anxiety, or depression over time. Others may cope by disengaging altogether, withdrawing from social settings or institutions that feel hostile or invalidating. While these responses are understandable and protective in the short term, they often come at the cost of mental clarity, self-worth, and communal connection. As one comprehensive review put it, strategies like chronic worry and emotion suppression, though used to survive the moment, can silently chip away at psychological resilience and overall well-being.[231]

Ultimately, these maladaptive behaviors are not signs of weakness but symptoms of a body overburdened biologically and socially. They reflect how African Americans have often had to adapt to an environment that remains racially toxic. Understanding these patterns is not at all about placing blame but expanding the context of a more informed narrative about how stress has been silently managed within the Black community. The compounded nature of this reality calls for greater self- and social compassion, community care, and access to culturally affirming wellness resources, all discussed more in Part IV of this book.

Conclusion

The lasting impact of the social inducers of chronic stress on African Americans cannot be overstated. From the enduring weight of systemic racism, Black communities have been forced to navigate a society that consistently undermines their safety, dignity, and well-being. These unrelenting stressors are not simply emotional burdens; they manifest biologically, driving persistent overactivation of stress pathways that damage health over time. The very structures designed to oppress have become engines of illness, embedding racial inequities into the physical bodies of those most harmed.

CHAPTER 5:
EPIGENETICS AND ANCESTRAL IMPRINTS: THE BIOLOGY OF INHERITED TRAUMA

Epigenetics, derived from the Greek word "epi," meaning "above," refers to the biological mechanisms that regulate gene activity without altering the DNA sequence. This developing field of science studies how environmental factors influence gene expression and explains how experiences can be biologically imprinted and passed down to future generations without altering the DNA sequence itself. Instead of direct genetic mutations, epigenetics involves chemical modifications to DNA and histone proteins, influencing how genes are expressed (meaning whether they are turned on or off). Traumatic experiences can trigger biological responses that are inherited, making descendants more prone to similar stress reactions, anxiety, or health vulnerabilities.

One of the most well-known experiments demonstrating how trauma can be passed down epigenetically was conducted on mice. Researchers trained male mice to fear a specific smell, acetophenone, which has a sweet, cherry-like scent, by pairing it with mild electric shocks. Over time, the mice learned to associate the smell with pain and exhibited strong fear responses whenever exposed to it, even without experiencing the shock.[232] When these mice later reproduced, their offspring, who had never been exposed to the shocks, also showed a fear response to the same smell. Even more remarkably, grand-offspring exhibited the same fear response, despite never having encountered the scent before. Upon further investigation, researchers found epigenetic changes in the sperm of the original mice, specifically in the gene responsible for detecting the acetophenone scent. These changes altered how their offspring's brains processed that smell, making them hypersensitive and primed to react with fear.[233] This mouse study offers more insight for researchers into beginning to understand what happens in human populations exposed to severe trauma, such as Jewish Holocaust survivors or communities that have endured long-term oppressive conditions, like enslaved Africans. The constant exposure to racial violence, discrimination, and chronic stress (as mentioned in the previous chapter) has likely shaped the biological stress responses of African Americans today, predisposing us to heightened levels of cortisol (the stress hormone), increased inflammation, and greater vulnerability to anxiety, depression, and PTSD.

Although human epigenetics is far more complex than a mouse model, this research provides a compelling biological explanation for why descendants of trauma survivors may struggle with stress-related health conditions at disproportionately high rates. The body remembers past traumas even if the mind does not, and epigenetic markers passed through generations may shape how individuals respond to stress, regulate emotions, and even develop chronic diseases. Epigenetics bridges the gap between nature and nurture, demonstrating that our lived experiences, both positive and negative, can leave biological imprints that influence not only our health but also the health of future generations. For populations subjected to prolonged trauma, such as enslaved Africans, epigenetics provides a robust framework for understanding how systemic oppression becomes biologically embodied, contributing to persistent health disparities. Understanding this science helps dismantle the false notion that health disparities in Black communities stem from a longstanding narrative of inherent biological inferiority. For populations subjected to sustained oppression, such as enslaved Africans and their descendants, epigenetics underscores how inequality is not only socially embedded but also biologically inherited.

Global Trauma Comparisons: Holocaust, Hunger, and Human Suffering

Historical trauma refers to the cumulative emotional, psychological, and physical effects of systemic oppression experienced by a group over time. Epigenetics offers a scientific explanation for how these experiences become biologically embedded. Stress, particularly chronic stress, is a key influencer of epigenetic changes. Chronic stress activates the body's hypothalamic-pituitary-adrenal (HPA) axis, releasing cortisol and other stress hormones that can cross the placenta and affect fetal brain development. All of which has led to studies revealing that maternal stress can influence the epigenetic markers of offspring. Prolonged activation of this system can alter gene expression, particularly in genes associated with stress regulation, immune function, and metabolism. Such alterations can also predispose offspring to heightened stress responses and anxiety.

Holocaust

The Holocaust (1933-1945) was a dark period in world history that involved a time of extreme brutality, including forced labor, starvation, medical experimentation, and mass executions, resulting in the death of approximately 6 million Jewish men, women, and children. This tragic era serves as a key case study for understanding how trauma influences epigenetic regulation. Neuroscientist Rachel Yehuda conducted research focusing on FKBP5 (a stress gene linked to PTSD, depression, and mood and anxiety disorders), and identified methylation changes in Holocaust survivors and their offspring.[234] Methylation is a process that regulates whether a gene is active or inactive by adding a methyl group to its DNA sequence. In Holocaust survivors, the FKBP5 intron 7 site exhibited a 10% higher level of methylation compared to a control group of Jewish individuals who lived outside Europe during World War II.[235] Interestingly, the children of survivors displayed a 7.7% lower methylation level at the same site compared to the control group.[236] These findings highlight an opposing direction in methylation patterns between survivors and their children.

According to Dr. John Krystal, a research psychiatrist, "children of traumatized parents are not simply born with a PTSD-like biology. They may inherit traits that promote resilience as well as vulnerability."[237] This dual inheritance reflects the complex interplay between adaptation and risk, where the biology of one generation adapts to its environment but may predispose the next generation to specific vulnerabilities. The biological consequences of these epigenetic changes were evident in the children of Holocaust survivors, who exhibited higher rates of anxiety and depression compared to the control group.[238] This study challenges the traditional notion that only direct experiences shape health outcomes. Instead, these findings demonstrate that the trauma endured by one generation can leave a biological imprint on subsequent generations, shaping their mental and physical health.

The findings from Holocaust survivor families provide a critical framework for understanding the epigenetic transmission of trauma in other historically oppressed populations, specifically African Americans. Dr. Yehuda validates this fact in an interview with the US Veterans Affairs, where she says there is nothing inherently "Jewish" about the phenomenon of how severe psychophysiological trauma can have intergenerational effects.[239] Enslaved Africans endured centuries of forced labor, family separations, and brutal punishments, traumas that mirror some of the extreme stressors faced by Holocaust survivors. The biological embedding of trauma, as seen in Holocaust research, helps explain how generations of African Americans may continue to experience heightened stress responses, increased inflammation, and greater risk for chronic diseases. Lastly, research collected on these Holocaust survivors provides a compelling scientific basis for why specific populations, as seen with African Americans, experience persistent health challenges rooted in ancestral suffering.

Dutch Hunger Winter

The Dutch Hunger Winter was a severe famine in the Netherlands during the winter of 1944-1945, near the end of World War II. The famine was caused by a German-imposed food blockade that drastically reduced food supplies to Dutch civilians. Over six months, an estimated 4.5 million people suffered from extreme malnutrition, with daily caloric intake dropping to as low as 400-800 calories per day, a fraction of what is necessary for survival. Thousands of people died from starvation and its complications. This enforced famine is recognized as a historical trauma, particularly because of its lasting biological effects on children who were in utero at the time.

Scientific studies on this atrocity revealed that timing was critical in determining the health effects of fetal malnutrition. Women who were in mid-to-late pregnancy during the famine gave birth to smaller babies with reduced birth weights. These infants, while underdeveloped at birth, had lower rates of obesity and cardiovascular disease later in life. Conversely, women exposed to famine during the first trimester of pregnancy gave birth to babies with more normal birth weights. However, these individuals grew up with higher rates of obesity, cardiovascular disease, and other metabolic disorders. Epigenetic analysis of the offspring's DNA revealed gene alterations linked to growth, metabolism, and stress regulation, particularly in IGF2, a gene crucial for fetal development.[240]

The results from the Dutch Hunger Winter underscore the concept of "fetal programming," where the intrauterine environment shapes the developmental trajectory of the fetus. A fetus exposed to a scarce environment adapts its metabolism to conserve energy, a mechanism that can become maladaptive in environments of abundance, leading to chronic diseases later in life. The epigenetic changes observed in the famine-exposed individuals persisted into adulthood and influenced their children's health, showing evidence of transgenerational effects.[241] This tragedy highlights the long-term health consequences of early environmental stressors and provides a context for understanding the epigenetic impact of the compounded stressors of systemic inequities.

The Dutch Hunger Winter study provides scientific evidence that severe nutritional deprivation during critical periods of fetal development can permanently alter gene expression, influencing how the body regulates metabolism, stress, and disease susceptibility across multiple generations. These findings closely parallel the experiences of enslaved African women and their descendants, many of whom endured chronic malnutrition, forced labor, and severe stress during pregnancy. In addition, this data yields global significance, particularly for understanding how intergenerational trauma and stress experienced by African Americans during enslavement and longstanding systemic oppression may contribute to modern-day health disparities.

New York African Burial Ground

Although there is no evidence of blood analysis collected from actual enslaved Africans to understand the cellular impact of their horrendous experience, scientists do have access to some of their skeletal remains left to tell the story. Discovered in the early 1990s in Lower Manhattan, the New York African Burial Ground is one of the most significant archaeological sites offering insight into enslaved Africans' lived experiences and health conditions in colonial America. Dating back to the 17th and 18th centuries, the burial site contained the remains of more than 15,000 African men, women, and children, revealing a disturbing narrative about the severe physical toll that enslavement inflicted upon their bodies. The skeletal remains provided irrefutable evidence of extreme labor, malnutrition, disease, and premature death, reinforcing what historical records have long suggested—that enslavement was a system of brutal physical exploitation that left lasting biological consequences.

Forensic examination of the skeletons showed extensive signs of physical wear and trauma. Many remains exhibited enlarged muscle attachment sites, a biological marker indicating that enslaved individuals were subjected to grueling, repetitive labor from early childhood until death.[242] Skeletal deformations, including lesions on the thigh bones and arthritis in the neck and back, provided further evidence of lifetimes spent carrying heavy loads and enduring physically punishing conditions. Child mortality rates among those interred at the burial ground were staggeringly high, with research indicating that 40% of the individuals buried there were children under the age of 12.[243] Infant deaths were particularly high, pointing to maternal malnutrition, disease exposure, and the hazardous conditions of childbirth for enslaved women. The presence of porotic hyperostosis, a condition linked to severe iron-deficiency anemia, in many of the remains demonstrated long-term nutritional deprivation and chronic stress. Malnutrition was further evidenced by dental enamel hypoplasia, a condition in which undernourished children develop thin, weakened enamel, making them more susceptible to tooth decay and infections. The mean age of death for those buried at the site was just 22.3 years, even lower than that of enslaved populations in Caribbean sugar plantations, where labor conditions were notoriously deadly. These early deaths were often attributed to untreated infections, extreme exhaustion, and cumulative stress that the body could no longer withstand.[244]

The short lives of those buried at the site are another indication that the biological toll of enslavement did not end with the individuals buried in the New York African Burial Ground; it likely influenced future generations through epigenetic changes. These findings reinforce a growing body of research demonstrating that historical trauma is not simply a social phenomenon but a biological one. Just as the Holocaust and Dutch Hunger Winter provided empirical evidence of transgenerational health effects, so too does the burial ground serve as a biological record of the enduring impact of slavery on African American health. While Holocaust survivors and Dutch famine survivors experienced extreme hardship over a shorter period, African Americans have endured over 400 years of violence, forced labor, systemic oppression, and discrimination that persist to this day. Extreme violence is traumatic for any duration of time; however, given the length and severity of our historical trauma, the biological impact on African Americans may be even more profound in its contribution to present-day racial health disparities.

The Blueprint Begins at Birth: Early Exposure and Lifelong Consequences

The National Institute of Environmental Health Sciences (NIEHS) is leading research into the Developmental Origins of Health and Disease (DOHaD)—a field that examines how exposures during sensitive periods of development, starting as early as conception and continuing through childhood, shape health outcomes later in life. These early-life exposures—whether nutritional deficiencies, environmental toxins, or psychosocial stressors—interact with both genetic and epigenetic factors to produce lasting biological effects. Sometimes, these changes can even be passed to future generations.

For African Americans, whose ancestral history includes the trauma of enslavement and whose present reality includes persistent systemic inequities, the DOHaD framework offers a critical lens for understanding racial health disparities. It provides a scientific explanation for how both historical trauma and current structural stressors contribute to disease vulnerability.

The DOHaD theory posits that many chronic conditions—including cardiovascular disease, Type II diabetes, asthma, reproductive disorders, and neurodegenerative diseases—have roots in early developmental windows, when organs and biological systems are still forming. During these sensitive stages, harmful exposures can disrupt normal development and alter biological pathways, increasing the likelihood of illness later in life.

NIEHS researchers emphasize that the impact of early exposures extends far beyond immediate health. These exposures can set the stage for long-term disease risk, especially in communities facing consistent environmental and social adversity. For African Americans, who disproportionately experience both the health conditions and the upstream drivers behind them, the DOHaD research underscores how deeply health inequities are embedded, not just in the social fabric, but in the biology shaped by that fabric across generations.

Moreover, the DOHaD research highlights how these effects can transcend generations. For instance, a mother's exposure to harmful environmental agents during pregnancy can alter the developmental trajectory of her child, with downstream effects on grandchildren. This concept aligns with epigenetic research previously discussed in this chapter, demonstrating that early-life exposures influence gene expression, perpetuating cycles of poor health across generations. The NIEHS has identified several conditions that are partly rooted in exposures occurring in the womb or during childhood, and they include:[245]

Cardiovascular Disease: Early-life nutritional deprivation or exposure to stress can disrupt the regulation of blood pressure and cholesterol, increasing the risk of hypertension and heart disease.

Obesity and Type II Diabetes: Maternal stress and poor nutrition during pregnancy can predispose offspring to metabolic dysregulation, leading to obesity and insulin resistance in adulthood.

Asthma: Exposure to air pollutants and other environmental toxins during childhood is strongly linked to higher rates of asthma, a condition that disproportionately affects Black children.

Behavioral Disorders and Neurodegenerative Diseases: Early-life stress and adverse social environments can alter brain development, increasing the risk of behavioral disorders like ADHD and mental health conditions such as depression and anxiety, as well as neurodegenerative diseases in later life.

Reproductive Disorders: Disruptions during critical developmental windows can lead to reduced fertility and other reproductive issues.

Certain Cancers: Early exposures to endocrine-disrupting chemicals or other toxins are associated with increased cancer risk.

These diseases are not only prevalent in African American communities. Still, they are often exacerbated by the same social determinants of health that drive early exposures, including poverty, environmental injustice, and systemic racism (previously discussed in Part II).

Environmental Exposures as Stressors

The burden of both historical and contemporary environmental exposures shapes the poor health outcomes of African Americans at a disproportionate rate. These exposures serve as stressors, compounding the physical, mental, and social health challenges faced by Black communities. Key environmental exposures, as pointed out by the NIEHS, along with their relevance to African American health (discussed further in Part II) include:[246]

1. Nutrition

Historically, enslaved Africans were subjected to severe nutritional deprivation, with diets limited to meager rations of cornmeal and fatty pork. This lack of dietary diversity and essential nutrients hindered growth and development and set the stage for future generations' metabolic disorders. Today, African Americans disproportionately live in food deserts, where access to fresh fruits, vegetables, and other healthy foods is limited. Barbie, a single mother in Philadelphia featured in ‹A Place at the Table,' struggled with food insecurity while raising two toddlers. Despite securing full-time employment, she lost eligibility for food assistance. Unfortunately, gainful employment ultimately widened the gap between her need for food and viable access, instead of the intended goal of closing it. This highlights how poverty, stress, and metabolic health are tightly linked. The persistence of food insecurity perpetuates cycles of poor nutrition and chronic diseases like obesity, diabetes, and hypertension.

2. Exogenous Toxins

The exposure of African Americans to environmental toxins has deep historical roots. During slavery, toxic work environments in plantations and industrial settings exposed enslaved people to hazardous substances. Today, many African Americans are more likely to live near industrial facilities, landfills, and highways, or work in toxic plants, leading to higher exposure to air pollutants and endocrine disruptors like plastics and pesticides. These toxins have been linked to asthma, cancer, and reproductive disorders, contributing to the high disease burden in Black communities.

3. Relationships and Social Dynamics

The systematic dismantling of African American families during slavery, through forced separations and the prohibition of cultural and familial practices, created a legacy of social disconnection. The lack of maternal nurturing and support compounded the stress of these fractured relationships. In contemporary times, Black families continue to face stressors such as mass incarceration, economic instability, and limited access to mental health resources, which perpetuate cycles of stress and adverse health outcomes. Families that do not face stressors related to socioeconomic inequality may deal with other stressors related to identity, belonging, and survivor's guilt.

4. Physical Locations and Access to Resources

The historical displacement of African Americans, from forced migration during slavery to segregation and redlining, has left lasting scars on Black communities. Many African Americans reside in neighborhoods with poor housing quality, limited healthcare facilities, and underfunded schools. These environmental conditions create chronic stress and limit access to the resources necessary for healthy development, perpetuating health disparities. For those not vulnerable due to housing, the tradeoff can come from conforming to less-than-welcoming environments. Maladaptive trauma responses become tools for survival among African Americans in the daily life experience of navigating neighbors, workplaces, and other environments where they do not feel safe enough or free enough to bring their guards down. What protects their emotional vulnerabilities and physical life can still come with cellular consequences of the engaged stress response.

PART III: THE BIOLOGY OF OPPRESSION

Scientific Reinforcements

Compelling studies specifically highlighting African Americans reiterate the DOHaD findings on the transgenerational health impact of the lived environment influences (also known as maternal stressors). To further capture how damaging navigating a race-based climate can be on the transgenerational health of African Americans, a pivotal study by David & Collins revealed some enlightening findings. Data collected indicated that the birth weights of first-generation African immigrants in the United States initially mirrored those of white Americans. However, by the second and third generations, birth weights among their descendants declined, converging toward those of African Americans. This trend starkly contrasts with the pattern observed among first-generation European immigrants, whose birth weights were similar to those of African Americans and then increased over successive generations to be more closely aligned with those of white Americans.

These findings provide compelling evidence that social and environmental factors, rather than genetic predisposition, drive racial disparities in birth outcomes.[247] The findings from David and Collins, as well as the CDC's analysis of birth outcomes (discussed in chapter 4), are clear indicators of the enduring legacy of systemic racism and social inequities. This study profoundly demonstrates that the American environment (racial climate) becomes increasingly disruptive to health for subsequent generations of African immigrants, while it is more beneficial for European immigrants. The persistent disparities in birth weight and preterm births among African Americans reflect the cumulative effects of historical trauma and contemporary oppression.

In addition, a study by Kuzawa and Sweet indicates that the cyclical nature of systemic inequities further exacerbates the transmission of stress-related health impacts. Generations of exposure to the same social-environmental risks as previous generations, such as poverty, limited access to quality healthcare, and environmental hazards, create a vicious cycle that perpetuates health disparities. They provide a basis for understanding this phenomenon as "environmentally responsive phenotypic plasticity." This term illustrates how social conditions can become biologically embodied, influencing gene expression and shaping health outcomes across generations due to an undisturbed, inequitable environment.[248] The sheer enormity of these stressors as recurring events creates not only a psychological burden on those living the experience but also a biological burden on those generations thereafter until the social cycle breaks the genetic predisposition.

Conclusion

As explored in this section, the chronic stress imposed by racism, socioeconomic inequality, and exclusionary practices has produced ongoing wear and tear on Black bodies, making them more vulnerable to diseases such as hypertension, diabetes, and heart disease. Yet, beyond these immediate effects, the science of epigenetics reveals an even more profound and more alarming truth: that the trauma of slavery, racial terror, and generational oppression has been biologically imprinted across time, leaving traces that still shape health outcomes today. Through the combined understanding of cross-cultural historical trauma, the demonstration of increased chronic disease susceptibility, and the research by the DOHaD, it paints a clear path around maternal health exposure and transgenerational cycles of disadvantage and disease. This current research also reveals evidence of how one woman is at least three generations walking. This includes the generation she belongs to and the unfertilized eggs she carries at birth, and inside those eggs is her genetic material that leaves an imprint not only on her child's development but also on what will one day evolve into reproductive cells that will produce her future grandchildren. As individualized as she is at birth, she represents three generations of herself. The environmental exposure she receives before her own birth and beyond will have a long-standing impact on her genetic line, just as the two preceding generations have had on her. Together, these insights expose the profound and enduring ways that historical and

PART III: THE BIOLOGY OF OPPRESSION

ongoing oppression continue to shape the health of African Americans, not only through lived experience but also through biological inheritance.

For guided discussion questions and activities, visit:
https://wellnessedu.blackcellconsulting.com
to access your FREE REFLECTION GUIDE.

Part IV:
RECLAIMING BLACK WELLNESS

Part IV: RECLAIMING BLACK WELLNESS

SO STRONG by Labi Stiffre

The higher you build your barriers
The taller I become
The further you take my rights away
The faster I will run
You can deny me, you can decide
To turn your face away

No matter 'cause there's
... Something inside so strong
I know that I can make it
Though you're doing me wrong, so wrong
You thought that my pride was gone, oh no
There's something inside so strong
Oh, something inside so strong

... The more you refuse to hear my voice
The louder I will sing
You hide behind walls of Jericho
Your lies will come tumbling
Deny my place in time, you squander wealth that's mine
My light will shine so brightly it will blind you

... Brothers and sisters
When they insist we're just not good enough
Well we know better
Just look him in his eyes and say
We're gonna do it anyway
We're gonna do it anyway
... There's something inside so strong
And I know that I can make it
Though you're doing me wrong, so wrong
You thought that my pride was gone, oh no
There's something inside so strong, oh
Something inside so strong

To speak of wellness in the African American community is to speak of something that has been systematically threatened, stolen, and undermined for generations. Wellness, true, holistic wellness that encompasses the mind, body, and spirit, has never simply been about diet, exercise, or annual checkups. For Black people in America, reclaiming wellness is a radical act of survival and self-determination. It is the deliberate process of restoring what was stripped away through centuries of violence, exploitation, and exclusion. When a community is continuously under siege by structural barriers that comprise every domain of life, wellness becomes more than just the absence of disease. Holding onto wholeness in the face of forces that seek to fracture you becomes a daily fight.

To reclaim wellness in such a context means pushing back against the systems and ideologies that have long worked to make Black suffering appear normal, inevitable, or deserved. It means naming harm, understanding its roots, and consciously choosing healing practices that restore balance to the individual and the community as a whole. It is acknowledging that the same society that pathologizes Blackness and ignores Black pain cannot be trusted to define or provide the truest sense of wellness. Therefore, reclaiming wellness requires creating new models grounded in cultural truth, ancestral wisdom, and collective care, where the goal is not merely to survive but to thrive, unapologetically.

In the final chapters ahead, we will explore what this reclamation looks like in practice. First, we will examine The Collectivism of Wellness, recognizing that healing for African Americans cannot exist in isolation. Family, community, and shared cultural identity are essential to any meaningful wellness strategy, offering support and strength against ongoing oppression. Next, we will turn to Individualized Wellness Practices, exploring personal strategies that center the unique needs of the Black body and mind, from stress reduction and nutrition to spiritual grounding and self-advocacy in healthcare spaces. Together, these approaches form a blueprint for how wellness can be reclaimed, nurtured, and passed onto future generations, according to our own values and terms defined for us, by us.

Part IV: RECLAIMING BLACK WELLNESS

CHAPTER 6:
THE COLLECTIVISM OF WELLNESS

For African Americans, the journey toward wellness has never been walked alone. Across generations, in the face of relentless oppression, collective strength has been the foundation of survival. The resilience of our ancestors, those who endured the unimaginable and still carved out moments of joy, healing, and connection, offers us a guiding light on what can often feel like a dark and uncertain path. Their wisdom teaches us that wellness is not solely an individual pursuit, but a shared responsibility and a communal inheritance. When the forces around us threaten to break the body and spirit, it is the power of community that sustains us.

The Collectivism of Wellness reimagines health not as a private or solitary achievement, but as something rooted in togetherness. It challenges the idea that wellness is only about personal discipline or individual self-care. Instead, it recognizes that true, lasting health and longevity come from collective action, cultural preservation, and mutual support. In this chapter, we will explore how community care, intergenerational wisdom, and shared cultural practices form the foundation of Black wellness, offering a pathway not just to survive oppressive systems but to thrive despite them.

Resilience as Resistance

The resilience of African Americans is a testament to an unbreakable spirit that has refused to submit to oppression, no matter how deeply it was embedded into the foundation of American society. From the moment enslaved Africans were forcibly taken from their homelands, they were thrust into a violent system of dehumanization designed to strip them of their identity and culture. Our ancestors resisted, not just through physical uprisings, but through their quiet yet radical acts of cultural preservation, storytelling, and faith. In the face of being socially and politically silenced, they passed down languages, traditions, and spirituals that spoke of freedom yet to come. Even after emancipation, when new barriers like Black Codes and Jim Crow laws arose, African Americans built schools, businesses, and entire communities that thrived despite systemic efforts to erase them. The intellectual and creative brilliance of Black leaders, from Reconstruction-era politicians to civil rights organizers, continuously met each new form of oppression with an even greater force of determination and strategy.

That same resilience continues today, as African Americans navigate a modern landscape still fraught with racial disparities in education, healthcare, and the justice system. The strategies have evolved, but the spirit remains the same. Movements like Black Lives Matter and grassroots activism echo the work of past generations, ensuring that demands for justice never fade. Black entrepreneurs, scholars, and artists push back against economic and cultural exclusion, crafting spaces where Black excellence flourishes on its own terms. Even in industries where representation was once an afterthought, Black professionals are rewriting the narrative, breaking barriers, and reshaping systems from within. Resilience is not just about survival; it is about transformation. Through every era, no matter how sophisticated the obstacles became, the ingenuity, strength, and collective power of African Americans rose to meet the challenge, proving time and time again that our legacy is one of endurance, innovation, and triumph.

The fact that oppressive barriers that have been strategically and structurally placed to deny African Americans an equitable opportunity to thrive in our whole health and well-being is irrefutable. Equal-

Part IV: RECLAIMING BLACK WELLNESS

ly indisputable are the remarkable strength and resilience that have kept us on the quest for new and increasingly innovative ways to maneuver past the insurmountable obstacles and challenges we face. Without this exceptional strength and resilience, the Black community would have had every legitimate excuse one could conceive of to give up hope, give up dreams of better days, if not for them, for the future generations that followed. Even with barriers in place at every turn, as a collective whole, the Black community is still standing. Some have gone on to truly thrive and soar, and many have learned to navigate the art of surviving while Black. At the end of the day, the community is not extinct. Black people are still here making our mark in the world in big and small ways, yet all significant.

Even while it is evident that African Americans have been able to withstand the Chicago "Hawk-like" forceful winds of anti-Black racism and all of its multi-layered oppressive expressions, imagine the accomplishments being exponentiated without those barriers in place. The achievements would be endless. Every human being is hard-wired for survival, but when Black people are required to bob and weave through discrimination, jump over racial hurdles, and keep their heads on a swivel while moving about oppressive environments, it strengthens survival skills. Skills are defined by the Britannica Dictionary as the ability to do something that comes from training, experience, or practice.

The truth is that discrimination has trained countless African Americans how to stand up and fight for Civil Rights and the multitude of injustices in this nation. Poverty has trained generations of African Americans how to acquire a dollar's worth of goods and resources from fifteen cents (a dime and a nickel) to provide for their families. Poverty has disciplined some African American students to rise at the crack of dawn to catch a city bus to attend high school far outside their neighborhood, participate in extracurricular activities, and work a part-time job out of necessity while maintaining A's & B's in hopes of getting accepted to a good college. Lack of representation in politics, science, business, literature, art, entertainment, and some sports has created a passion for many African Americans to break down the barriers of exclusion and pave a chiseled path towards entry not only for them but also to inspire the generations who would come after them. A hard-knock life has trained many young African American men and women to collapse the pain and challenges of their life experiences into rhythmic expressions laid over really tight beats. Even being too poor to afford instruments, some found a way to use even their mouths and hand claps to create a flow of beats and sounds that helped give birth to a hip-hop culture that has completely transformed the world.

Without barriers, survival skills can conveniently be repurposed into skills for thriving. For too long, the focus has been on the deficits that exist within the Black race. As long as they are viewed as deficits, the Black population will continue to not reach a higher collective level of achievement. It is not enough for only a small percentage to thrive and truly soar in their lives; the capacity to live up to one's highest potential is within everyone. Unfortunately, the art of surviving while Black can be downright tiring to the point where there is nothing left to give any other aspect of our lives, including our personal health. The many faces of oppression are relentless, and it wears us out physically, emotionally, and psychologically, but somehow, African Americans manage to rise to meet the challenges of a brand-new day, every day. That is not a deficit. Out of necessity, Black people have actually created a surplus of resilience and strength. The not-so-good news is that the body craves balance, so the problem with too much of a good thing is that it takes the body out of natural homeostasis.

An example of this would be a car that is designed to go 160 miles per hour would probably not make it very far at persistent maximum speed. Forget about that road trip from California to New York, cars need time to allow the engine to cool down. Although the engine may have the horsepower to achieve that speed, endurance is still pivotal. When the car is manufactured, everything else about the car should equate in endurance levels to match the high speed.

This would include the durability of the tires, the exhaust releasing the fumes from combustion, the fuel burning rate and storage capacity, and the overall weight and quality of the auto body frame materials to withstand the power and force of such rapid movement. Not to mention sturdy brake pads that allow the vehicle to come to a complete stop as needed. Therefore, it becomes more than a matter of speed capacity but also maintenance of the load and sustainability over time at those higher-performance levels; otherwise, the car will crash and burn.

Just like the car, if we equate resilience in the human body to horsepower, we are not designed to perpetually exist in a state of resilience and strength. Both require extended periods of rest, relaxation, and recovery. In addition, sustainability and survivability rates increase when all other components of the human body are conditioned to meet higher levels of resilience and strength, such as a healthy heart and a strong immune system. Otherwise, like the car that overheats, the body can more quickly become overwhelmed to the point of physical and emotional burnout. This is where building a skill set to support personal health determinants becomes very important. Equipping the body with more life-giving tools on a daily and consistent basis will help mitigate the long-term health impact of the structural barriers built for our demise. In unison African Americans can more proudly proclaim to face our oppressors, "AND STILL WE RISE!"

Mitigating Harm Through Community

The question is, who do we as African Americans have to become to live a healthier version of ourselves in the midst of pervasive racial toxicity and the barriers attached to it?

At the baseline of health is first understanding why it even matters in the first place. Our health matters because we matter and we always have. Society has imposed a negative tape on the Black community that reiterates in various forms that our lives do not matter. In Chapter 3 of this book, I pointed out the various forms of psychological dehumanization imposed upon our ancestors. The residual impact of the terror inflicted upon their minds conditioned them towards more division and individualized hopelessness of freedom. Undoubtedly so, the psychological chains of slavery have left an unhealed scarring beyond physiology and into self and community identity, as pointed out by Na'im Akbar in *Chains and Images of Psychological Slavery*. As difficult as it may be to read about the brutalities of slavery, it is still a history that occurred and continues to subconsciously influence our own behavior and how we interact with our oppressive environment, ourselves, and one another. Healing comes first with acknowledgement and practicing an intentionality from within to produce not just a counter narrative but a counter outcome of the premature death and disease we see rampant in our communities. Otherwise, it becomes easy to get stuck in a plight of perpetual stages of survival, without ever crossing the threshold to transformation.

Every person on the planet was created to do great things, whatever that means for them. "Great" does not mean "famous" or "celebrity," but it does mean fully expressing a divine birthright to live out meaningful purpose and potential. The health and well-being of each of us matter because the physical body serves as the conduit for our gifts, talents, and contributions to the world to manifest as an offering to humanity. Unhealed minds and bodies do more to limit participation in the advancement of self and community while making survival look more like a form of entrapment rather than a celebration of existence. Mitigation of dis-ease within the mind and body begins from the relationship we have to the one true Source of creation, also known as God (and called by many other names), which is a reflection of the relationship we have with ourselves. Despite all of the societal messages and barriers in place to consistently remind us that we have no significant value in comparison to our white counterparts, to know God is to know the mere fact that we exist, automatically gives us immeasurable value and worth. To be disconnected from the spiritual aspect of ourselves makes us vul-

Part IV: RECLAIMING BLACK WELLNESS

nerable to being conditioned by society and the internal battlefield attached to it. However, to live from the source of power found in knowing God is to build a life where obstacles and challenges are not limiting us but lifting us. This is by no means an easy task, but it is definitely achievable. Just like the story of the donkey who fell into the bottom of a dry well and was meant to be buried there by the owner who thought he was not worth saving, with each shovel of dirt that fell upon him, he shook it off his back, and it fell underneath his feet. As the dirt piled into the well, he was able to take another step up and up until he finally reached the top. The same dirt meant to bury him gave him a route of escape, therefore saving his life.

After emancipation, our ancestors were released into an environment of legal freedom but also designed to bury them slowly with structural oppression and social hostility. Instead of succumbing to unfair treatment, inequitable access, and an outright refusal towards them integrating into white-dominated institutions, they shook the dirt off their backs. Without any wealth whatsoever and being excluded from economic opportunities or political participation, African Americans turned to one another to survive and ultimately thrive. The very communities once bound by the trauma of enslavement became the foundation for a collective transformation. Mutual aid societies, Black churches, and cooperative economic efforts emerged as lifelines. These were not merely cultural or religious centers; they became hubs of education, business, childcare, healthcare, and activism. The necessity of survival brought them back to a level of interdependence that their African ancestors had known.

Collective resilience during post-emancipation reverberated across many sectors of Black life in America as they learned to expand in the fullness of living as free human beings. The Negro Motorist Green Book, published annually beginning in 1936 by Victor Hugo Green, was a literal roadmap for Black travelers to safely navigate a segregated and often dangerous America, providing a network of Black-owned hotels, restaurants, and gas stations when mainstream establishments would not serve them. Black schools, established under segregation and often funded by the community itself, like the Rosenwald Schools across the South, were beacons of education and hope despite inadequate public support. Similarly, entertainment venues such as the Chitlin' Circuit provided platforms for Black performers when white-owned venues barred their entry, nurturing legends like Aretha Franklin and James Brown. These examples underscore how African Americans not only resisted marginalization but also created thriving cultural and economic ecosystems. Their survival and flourishing was a communal act of transformation rooted in unity, resourcefulness, and a shared vision of dignity and progress. During the post-Civil Rights Era, the Black community, for the first time, had options of collectivism or individualism. With the pressure of conformity and the risk of being further alienated from mainstream society, unfortunately, the latter grew into a more dominant choice over time. The current social and political climate, with its "Make America Great Again" mantra, is reawakening a necessity for the same interdependence our ancestors utilized as a key essential for creating healing and transformation within the community today.

COLLECTIVE HEALTH & WELL-BEING

The ethnocentric-monocultural value system of American society leads African Americans to believe that health, like everything else, is an individual journey that can only be achieved by the hard work and dedication of the individual. For marginalized groups such as African Americans living in an already oppressed environment, embracing such individualistic concepts as this can become more destructive to health and well-being than beneficial. To honor our strong, brave, courageous, and resilient ancestors, let's consider embracing the same approach they used to get ahead…collectivism. That begins with embodying the African Proverb, "If you want to get there fast, go alone. If you want to get far, go together." The experience of life will always taste sweeter when it is shared within a community of support.

During the Jim Crow Era, segregation birthed a need to demonstrate what we would label today as The Nguzo Saba, otherwise known as the 7 Principles of Kwanzaa into a way of life. At that time, it was just a natural way our Black ancestors learned to navigate life successfully despite oppressive conditions. Today, celebrating the holiday of Kwanzaa from December 26 to January 1 has reached a more widespread recognition since its inception in 1966 by Maulana Ron Karenga. Nonetheless, the principles should not just be observed during the holiday season but embraced as a current way of life through daily intentional practices. Why is this important in relation to health and well-being? Health is a very private matter, how people choose to take care of themselves and participate in activities that are either supporting health and well-being or destroying it is up to that individual. At the end of the day, the individual will be the person most severely affected by the outcome of their health behaviors. Most can all agree with that statement. However, that type of limited thinking and understanding will not yield optimized results of an improved individual or collective achievement of wellness. As a community, we are only as strong as our weakest link. The historical trauma inflicted on the lived Black experience did not just impact individuals; it impacted whole communities and ultimately generations of us. Individual healing must be a collective effort, as all African Americans work together towards the healing of generations to come. "Each one, teach one" through love, support, and accountability.

Lastly, creating community and practicing collective care among African Americans is not only a cultural and historical act of resilience—it is also a scientifically supported path toward physiological healing. Research has shown that telomeres, the protective caps at the ends of our chromosomes (discussed in Chapter 4), are longer in individuals who experience strong social connections and a deep sense of belonging. According to Dr. Elizabeth Blackburn, Nobel Prize-winning scientist, and Dr. Elissa Epel, a health psychologist, social isolation and chronic stress, often the result of racialized experiences, contribute to the shortening of telomeres, accelerating aging and increasing the risk for disease. In contrast, according to their research, social cohesion and feeling a sense of safety within their neighborhoods has a protective effect on telomere shortening.[249] This means that the act of building an intentional Black community, rooted in shared cultural identity, mutual care, and collective power, can extend our healthspan at the cellular level. When we as African Americans come together to create safe, affirming spaces, whether through spiritual communities, family networks, wellness circles, or cultural coalitions, we engage in a form of resistance that heals the mind, body, and spirit. Individualized thinking, though often a survival strategy, cannot provoke the systemic cellular changes needed to heal from the compounded trauma of racial oppression. Healing, therefore, must be communal. In a system that thrives on division and internalized inferiority in us, togetherness is not only a radical act, it is a biological necessity. More than ever, we need to create our own spaces that allow us to belong, because belonging helps us live fully, not simply survive.

The African concept of Ubuntu states that "I am because we are." It was later expanded by African theologian John Mbiti to include "...and since we are, therefore I am." Ubuntu speaks to the heart of a cyclical pattern of connection that we must all honor in order to truly break the barriers to our wellness. Our community of belonging shapes and nurtures each individual, and as the individual grows and shares their gifts and talents with the community, everyone benefits from the presence and contribution of one another. The health and well-being of a community supports and nurtures the health and well-being of individuals. As individuals establish an optimized life, they are more fully equipped to be a beneficial presence to their community, and the cycle of wellness continues.

Collectivism is what will individually anchor us in a community of support that builds our resistance against narratives designed to destroy us from the inside outward, and instead, together, we can strengthen our resilience to rise from fighting to survive to thriving.

Part IV: RECLAIMING BLACK WELLNESS

Our ability to survive treacherous conditions has already been proven; now it is time to exercise the momentum of the community to enhance our lives. When we embrace the concept of health and well-being from a place of nurturing first, that is, internal self-talk, the relationship we have with ourselves is often shaped by the relationships we have with others, and vice versa. To live in an environment rich with empowerment, cultural affirmation, and accountability is foundational to optimizing individualized tools and strategies. Together the two components more powerfully create a cycle of healing where everyone benefits from and contributes to the growth and expansion of others.

History as well as contemporary times has already shown us that the upward mobility of the Black community is not a priority to the powers that be, which makes it even more imperative that it is a priority to us as a people individually and collectively. Together we can mobilize to improve our communities to whatever extent is possible, no more blaming, no more waiting; it is time for deliberate, intentional action towards healing ourselves through healing our communities. Doing for ourselves does not release the local and federal governments from the responsibility of firm legislation and economic investment to create a more equitable experience for African Americans. Nonetheless, in my best Iyanla Vanzant voice, I must say, "in the meantime," we got our own work to do. The way has already been paved, and the examples have already been shown to us by our ancestors who came out of slavery with nothing. No resources like we have today, no access to education like we have today, no comforts of home or material pleasures like what we have today. They had a deeply entrenched spiritual connection to God, physical strength, and mental endurance, all being fueled by a driving motivation to succeed at physical freedom, and they DID! The wheel does not need to be recreated; together, we can duplicate or enhance it for the benefit of the wider collective.

Just as there was a historical cultural erasure when our ancestors were forced to migrate into America, there are currently deliberate acts of historical erasure of the injustice done to them. The very act to erase them is another devaluation of us, our history, and our culture. We are living in a time where we cannot afford to leave the history of our people in the hands of others. Our history and our present-day health are deeply intertwined; to deny acknowledgement through erasure is a denial of its foundational role in most aspects of our current vulnerability to chronic disease. It is up to us to create deliberate acts of empowerment through education in our journey towards cultural and cellular healing for ourselves and, more importantly, the generations to come.

THE NGUZO SABA (7 PRINCIPLES OF KWANZAA) AS A FRAMEWORK FOR WELLNESS EMPOWERMENT

PRINCIPLE ONE:
UMOJA (UNITY)

Umoja, meaning unity, is the foundational principle of Kwanzaa, emphasizing the importance of togetherness in family, community, and the broader African diaspora. Historically, unity has been the bedrock of Black survival and resilience. From the Underground Railroad to the Civil Rights Movement, the collective strength of the African American community has always been central to overcoming systemic oppression. Enslaved Africans built kinship networks despite being forcibly separated from their biological families, creating fictive kin relationships where people bonded as brothers, sisters, and elders to preserve cultural identity and emotional stability.

In contemporary times, however, social fragmentation due to systemic barriers such as mass incarceration, economic disparity, and gentrification threatens the unity that once defined Black communities. Despite these challenges, grassroots social justice organizations such as Black Lives Matter and community-based healing initiatives reinforce the necessity of unity in addressing racial trauma and collective health disparities.

Impact on Holistic Health

Mental & Emotional Health:

Unity fosters a strong support system, which is crucial for mental well-being. Research shows that individuals with strong social support experience lower levels of depression.[250] For African Americans, unity helps buffer against the negative effects of racial stress and discrimination. The concept of communal coping, where individuals share burdens and provide mutual encouragement, has long been a survival mechanism in Black culture.

Physical Health:

Strong community ties correlate with better physical health outcomes. Studies indicate that social isolation increases the risk of chronic diseases, including hypertension and cardiovascular disease, both of which disproportionately affect African Americans.[251] Community-based fitness initiatives, like group exercise programs in Black churches or neighborhood running clubs, promote both physical health and social bonding.

Spiritual Health:

Umoja aligns deeply with African spiritual traditions that emphasize interdependence and the interconnectedness of all life. Many African cultural belief systems share that healing comes through the collective, whether through ancestral veneration, group prayers, or communal rituals. In Black churches today, collective worship and shared spiritual practices continue to be a source of healing and resilience.

Community Health:

The social determinants of health, such as: housing, education, and employment, are directly influenced by the strength of communal ties. When communities are unified, they have greater political power to advocate for better resources, fight against environmental racism, and demand equitable policies. The history of Black townships such as Rosewood and Black Wall Street shows how unity built thriving economies, while the destruction of such communities through systemic violence reveals how disunity weakens collective health.

Practical Applications for Umoja in Daily Life

Strengthen Family Bonds: Make an intentional effort to maintain family relationships, hold regular check-ins, and support each other emotionally. Bring back regular Sunday dinners, "Big Mama" style, which means that everyone feels welcomed at the table. Hosting a regular game night also helps you connect while having and creating new memories.

Engage in Community Activities: Where we live and play must matter to us first and foremost. Your presence alone speaks volumes, and your individual and collective voice reverberates even louder when we show up to volunteering with organizations and local activities that uplift the people, we are demonstrating a community showing up to support one another. This can also be done by attending neighborhood meetings to stay informed and work on residential solutions.

Prioritize Collective Healing: Something transformative happens when people who are hurting emotionally, physically, and spiritually find themselves in a comfortable and welcoming space. No judgment, no rejection, but a sense of belongingness that helps you feel safe enough to openly process the internal pain that racial trauma causes. These spaces can look like group therapy facilitated by a mental health counselor, church support groups, cultural healing circles, or after hours at the barber/beauty shops.

Support Black-Owned Businesses: Economic unity is a form of resistance. The financial success and sustainability of a Black-owned business is not only an individual win for the business but a collective win for us all. When we spend with Black businesses, we are communicating with our dollars that we find value in the goods and services they provide for us, and we value the opportunity to contribute towards the longevity of their business. This interchangeable relationship works optimally as long as owners demonstrate that they value the opportunity to meet the needs of the community with its goods and services.

Create Intergenerational Ties: Preserving wisdom, knowledge, traditions, and cultural pride must be passed on from the elder to the younger generations through intentional encounters. This can encourage youth to participate in direct mentorship programs. Pre-arranged "Elder Playdates" is another option used to create a bridge between the young and the old. These should involve activities where elders can interweave storytelling into the activity, designed to enhance youths' understanding of history and culture. Playdates to consider are cooking, gardening, scavenger hunts, or reading and discussing book passages, quotes, or picture books documenting history.

Umoja is more than just a principle; it is the lifeblood of collective well-being that courses through our veins. We were created to be social creatures. Whether through mental and emotional support, physical wellness, spiritual grounding, or community activism, unity provides the foundation for health and longevity in Black communities. Without unity, the strength to resist oppression and build sustainable, thriving communities weakens. Just like Big Mama Joe from "Soul Food" the movie reminded us, "one finger won't make an impact, but you ball all those fingers into a fist and you can strike a mighty blow." By embracing Umoja, we can reclaim the collective power necessary to heal, to grow, and to thrive.

PRINCIPLE TWO:
KUJICHAGULIA (SELF-DETERMINATION)

Self-determination, or Kujichagulia, is the principle of defining, naming, creating, and speaking for ourselves rather than being defined by others. It is a direct counter to the historical and contemporary forces that have attempted to strip African Americans of our autonomy, culture, and power. Self-determination has played a pivotal role in Black survival, from the resistance of enslaved Africans who fought against their captors to the Black Power Movement of the 1960s that called for cultural pride and political self-sufficiency.

Historically, enslaved Blacks were denied the right to make even the most basic decisions about their lives, from what to eat to whom they could marry. Yet resistance movements such as the Underground Railroad and Nat Turner's Rebellion in 1831 revealed that our ancestors chose their own fate and rather than allow it to be decided for them by their enslavers. Although laws such as the Black Codes and Jim Crow segregation reinforced this lack of agency well after slavery ended, Marcus Garvey's Back-to-Africa Movement exemplified how self-determination will always be an integral part of Black liberation.

In contemporary times, the media is a crucial element in how the Black narrative is told. Upholding Kujichagulia in journalism ensures that African Americans are seen and defined on our own terms, shaping a future informed by truth rather than stereotypes. Black journalism platforms such as Roland Martin and those on the Black Star Network have reclaimed the narrative about black life, history, politics, and issues from mainstream media's often distorted lens. They have created a medium for their own voices as representatives of the community to tell unfiltered, authentic stories in an act of empowerment and resistance against misrepresentation as well as underrepresentation of Black joy and magic.

Impact on Holistic Health

Mental & Emotional Health:

When individuals are able to define themselves, they experience higher self-esteem and psychological resilience. Research shows that a strong sense of self-esteem protects against depression and anxiety.[252] The lack of self-determination, on the other hand, can lead to lower self-esteem and internalized oppression, where negative societal narratives become part of one's self-perception, contributing to stress and self-doubt.

Physical Health:

Self-determination extends to the ability to make informed health decisions and advocate for one's medical care. A major issue in Black health disparities is medical racism, where Black patients' concerns are dismissed or undertreated. Self-advocacy in these spaces is a form of resistance. We have the right to assert that our lives matter to us, even more so in medical spaces that are designated to improve our health and well-being and not minimize our need for care.

Spiritual Health:

Self-determination allows individuals to reclaim spiritual practices that were stripped away through colonization and forced conversion. Many African Americans are returning to traditional African spirituality, engaging in ancestral veneration, the use of plant-based medicines, and other holistic healing practices that align with our cultural heritage. This spiritual autonomy offers a deep sense of empowerment and holistic healing.

Community Health:

The principle of Kujichagulia is seen in Black-led organizations that push for policy changes in housing, education, and criminal justice. It is also evident in the Buy Black movement, which seeks to reduce economic dependence on white-owned businesses that are not reinvesting in Black communities. This shifts the focus towards fostering environments of Black entrepreneurship and self-sufficiency.

Practical Applications for Kujichagulia in Daily Life

Own Your Narrative: Escaping a sea of negative stereotypes can sometimes be daunting. Be intentional about defining yourself and your identity. Who do you say you are? Replace any negative attributes with positive parallels and repeat them to yourself in the form of affirmations until you believe them, embrace them, and embody them. Replacement examples include Fearful = I am courageous; Unattractive = I am beautiful/handsome; Poor = I am abundant; Stupid = I am brilliant. When you need help remembering who you really are, and we all do sometimes, seek out spaces that affirm Black excellence and culture.

Advocate for Your Health: Your body is always communicating with you; therefore, it is your job to not only listen to its needs for attention and care but to not stop until those concerns are addressed in a way that you experience some level of relief. There is relief in knowing what the medical problem is and an even greater relief when the condition is effectively treated. Feel empowered to be the voice of your body by respectfully speaking up in medical settings, asking questions when you need more understanding, seeking second opinions if necessary, and being proactive in regular self-care.

Embrace Cultural Expression: Beyond looking good in your freshly styled crowns and stellar threads, wearing natural hair and cultural clothing is a statement of pride, a celebration of Black identity. Also, purchase beautiful Black art and other cultural adornments to decorate your home and other sacred spaces. Regularly play some vibratory beats that compel your hips to swing and your feet to move. These are cultural traditions that will reinforce your warm embrace of African American pride.

Support Black-Owned Businesses: Economic self-determination is crucial to independence and generational wealth-building.

Put your money where your mouth is. Build the collective empowerment of "for us, by us" through spending your dollars with businesses that were designed with the needs of the Black community in mind and supporting its initiatives.

Engage in Civic Action: National elections definitely matter, but you will feel a direct impact in local politics even more significantly. Your voice matters, and your vote matters. Community organizing helps to get your voice and your concerns heard in policy advocacy around issues impacting your own backyard. Collectively, we have the power to put officials on the ballot and elect those who represent our interest. Change begins to unfold when you show up at the meeting.

Kujichagulia is about reclaiming power—power over identity, health, and community. By rejecting imposed definitions and embracing autonomy, African Americans can reshape our narrative and strengthen collective well-being. It is up to us to define ourselves, name ourselves, and speak for ourselves, instead of being defined and spoken for by others. Angela Davis reminds us that, "I am no longer accepting the things I cannot change. I am changing things I cannot accept." The power to strengthen our communities ultimately lies within each of us that creates the larger collective body.

PRINCIPLE THREE:
UJIMA (COLLECTIVE WORK AND RESPONSIBILITY)

Ujima, meaning collective work and responsibility, is the principle that underscores the interconnectedness of the African American experience. It reflects the idea that one person's well-being is tied to the well-being of the collective, emphasizing that communal care and shared responsibility are essential for survival and progress. This principle has long been the foundation of Black resilience to rise above systemic injustices affecting our community. Historically, African Americans have relied on communal survival strategies to navigate centuries of oppression. Today, this principle is just as relevant in tackling health disparities, economic instability, and racial trauma.

During slavery, enslaved Africans engaged in collective parenting, where the entire community participated in raising and protecting children to the best of their ability, knowing that biological families could be torn apart at any moment. This tradition of "other mothering" where grandmothers, aunts, and unrelated women cared for children was a direct embodiment of Ujima, ensuring that no child was left without love and guidance. Post-emancipation, African Americans built mutual aid organizations to provide financial assistance to those in need of sick care, burials, job training, education, and other community needs. On college campuses around the country, Black fraternities and sororities, collectively referred to as the Divine Nine, were formed to not only foster personal excellence but also collectively build kinship, racial pride, civic action, and participate in various forms of community service. Throughout the Civil Rights Movement, Ujima was the driving force behind boycotts, sit-ins, and political organizing, demonstrating how collective action could dismantle oppressive systems.

In contemporary times, Ujima is evident in grassroots movements like Black Lives Matter, which calls for collective responsibility in addressing police violence and systemic racism. Food sovereignty projects such as the Soul Fire Farm demonstrate a commitment to ending food apartheid through a process that supports social and ecological transformation. In addition, the rise of Black-led community health initiatives such as the Barbershop Quartet Health Outreach Program makes health screening available in this non-traditional wellness space, and the use of local mental health healing circles further illustrates how Ujima remains a pillar of Black survival and wellness.

Impact on Holistic Health

Mental & Emotional Health:

The psychological benefits of communal support are well-documented. Studies show that strong social networks reduce stress and the risk of depression.[253] Black communities that prioritize collective healing spaces, such as therapy groups and faith-based counseling, experience lower levels of racial trauma-related distress.[254] The burden of racialized experiences can be isolating, but Ujima fosters a shared emotional resilience, ensuring that no one struggles alone.

Physical Health:

Health disparities in Black communities, including higher rates of diabetes, hypertension, and maternal mortality, are often tied to social determinants of health.[255] Community-based health programs, like free mobile clinics and fitness groups, serve as modern expressions of Ujima, allowing Black individuals to take collective responsibility for their well-being. Exercise groups in predominantly Black spaces, like local church walking groups, foster a sense of community and accountability, improving health outcomes.

Spiritual Health:

Many African cultures view health as holistic and communal, where healing is not just individual but collective. Spiritual traditions such as group prayers, healing circles, and community-based wellness practices reinforce the idea that well-being is shared.

Black churches and mosques continue to serve as spiritual healing and advocacy centers, providing spiritual and material support to those in need.

Community Health:

The power of community-driven solutions is seen in Black-led organizations addressing food insecurity, housing instability, and financial literacy. Groups like Black Urban Growers (BUGs) promote food sovereignty, ensuring that Black communities have access to fresh, culturally appropriate foods. Mutual aid funds, which redistribute wealth and resources within Black communities, are a modern embodiment of Ujima, directly challenging economic disparities.

Practical Applications for Ujima in Daily Life

Support Black-Led Community Initiatives: Show up as the living embodiment of the resource for your local organizations. All it takes is the regular dedication and willingness to serve, from the administrative offices to keeping the facilities clean, organized, and stocked with snacks. Whether you have advanced skills, low skills, or no skills, there is a place for you to contribute your time and energy in organizations focused on education, health, and economic development.

Build Support Networks: Acknowledging the benefits of community is the first step towards finding your tribe. The journey of health and wellness is more enjoyable when shared with those working on similar goals. Join or create groups centered on wellness, whether through fitness clubs, spiritual fellowships, or mental health circles. Social media sites such as local Facebook groups and Meetup.com can also serve as resources to find or build these networks.

Share Knowledge and Resources: Find creative ways to give back to your community with your time, talents, or tithes by seeking out people who can be the best benefactor of your resources.

That can look like teaching the neighborhood boys and girls how to change a tire or hiring youth in your neighborhood to complete tasks involving technology, chores, and organizing. All of which can foster healthy growth and interactions while building a stronger community.

Participate in Local Activism: Advocate for policies that improve healthcare access, environmental justice, and economic equity in Black neighborhoods.

Practice Communal Healing: Engage in intergenerational dialogue by creating small and large group circles for all ages to discuss issues impacting the community from the perspective of their represented age group. This provides everyone with opportunities to learn from each other and feel valued, seen, and respected for what they have to share at these church, cultural, or social sponsored events.

Ujima is the foundation of Black collective strength. It teaches that healing, progress, and justice are not individual pursuits, but communal responsibilities. By applying this principle, as African Americans we can reclaim agency over our health, advocate for one another, and disrupt the cycles of oppression that threaten community wellness. As Audre Lorde famously said, "Without community, there is no liberation." Ultimately, the obligation of freedom falls on us.

PRINCIPLE FOUR:
UJAMAA (COOPERATIVE ECONOMICS)

Ujamaa, meaning cooperative economics, is the principle that emphasizes shared financial growth, economic self-sufficiency, and community-based wealth-building. Collective empowerment is bred by ownership and harnessing control over the types of goods and services distributed to its community and by whom. This principle of Ujamaa challenges the economic disenfranchisement that has historically restricted Black prosperity and underscores the necessity of collective economic empowerment as a strategy for improving overall health and well-being. Former educator Dr. Barbara Sizemore reminded us that true empowerment comes from ownership and the ability to dictate what is sold, consumed, and valued within our own communities. This requires rejecting the destructive pattern that has been normalized and beginning to redesign our own culture rooted in self-determination rather than dependency.[256] We have always had the capacity to exercise this power, but there has been an intentionality to suppress it with distractions of moment-to-moment survival.

Historically, Black communities have practiced Ujamaa through mutual aid societies, Black-owned businesses, and economic initiatives prioritizing group prosperity over individual wealth. The destruction of self-sufficient Black communities like Tulsa's Black Wall Street (1921) and Rosewood (1923) was not just an economic attack but a holistic health catastrophe, as it robbed entire populations of financial security, communal pride, and stable living conditions. Today, economic disparities continue to manifest in lower wages, fewer job opportunities, and wealth gaps (discussed previously in Part II), all of which directly impact health outcomes for African Americans.

Throughout history, African Americans have worked to build economic independence despite systemic barriers. During the Reconstruction era, formerly enslaved Black people pooled their resources to buy land, establish businesses, and create thriving communities. Today, we have organizations such as the Freedom Georgia Initiative, an economic co-op that was established in 2020 to reintroduce a for us, by us safe haven for Black families to live and thrive in spite of the treacherous past of the United States. History has repeatedly demonstrated how Black economic progress has been met with structural violence, from racially motivated massacres to the federal government's refusal to support Black farmers and business owners. The racial wealth gap remains one of the largest obstacles to Black health equity, as economic stability is directly tied to access to quality healthcare, nutritious food, and safe living environments.

Impact on Holistic Health

Mental & Emotional Health:

Reports from the American Psychological Association in 2020 indicate that financial stress is one of the leading causes of anxiety and depression. For Black Americans, financial strain is often compounded by discriminatory economic policies that limit access to high-paying jobs and capital for business development. Wealth-building through cooperative economics provides a sense of financial security, reducing chronic stress and promoting mental well-being.

Physical Health:

Studies show that economic instability contributes to poor health outcomes, including higher rates of hypertension, diabetes, and heart disease.[257] A lack of health insurance and disposable income often means less access to preventative care and delayed treatment. Investing in Black-owned businesses, particularly those that focus on health and wellness, ensures that money stays within the community and contributes to resources geared towards improving the health outcomes of the community through sponsorships and other initiatives.

Spiritual Health:

Many African spiritual traditions emphasize collective prosperity over individual wealth. Economic empowerment that benefits the entire community aligns with these ancestral values and promotes a sense of purpose and shared success. Supporting Black businesses and entrepreneurs is a spiritual act of reclamation, ensuring that wealth is circulated within the community instead of being extracted by external forces.

Community Health:

Economic power directly influences housing conditions, educational opportunities, and healthcare access. When Black communities own their businesses, banks, and grocery stores, they can ensure higher-quality resources for their residents. Food deserts and healthcare deserts are direct results of economic disinvestment in Black communities. By practicing cooperative economics, African Americans can advocate for and fund initiatives that bring essential services to these neglected areas.

Practical Applications for Ujamaa in Daily Life

Support Black-Owned Businesses: Our daily, weekly, and monthly lives involve countless transactions; make a positive difference to Black businesses by being intentional in your effort to use them for some of those goods and services. This can include restaurants, retail outlets, banks, and professional services. In the event you do not live near local BOBs, there are Black Business Directories and other online national listings of resources for the culture available.

Participate in Group Economics: Combined dollars have the ability to acquire more and at a faster rate than individual efforts towards building financial independence. Form investment groups, cooperatives, or community savings plans to pool resources for business development and property ownership. In 2020 Nineteen Black families pooled together their resources to purchase 97 acres of land; as of 2021 it quickly grew to 502 acres, which they have been using to build healthy, sustainable Black communities.

Teach Financial Literacy: Frederick Douglass reminds us that "it is easier to raise strong children than to repair broken adults."[258]

Perpetual financial distress can leave one feeling not just broke in the pockets but broke in the spirit as well. Exposing our children and young adults to education on budgeting, credit management, savings, and investing helps break cycles of economic hardship and sets them up for a greater chance at financial success at an earlier age. Buy a few stocks in one of their favorite clothing brands and teach them how to monitor it and compare the growth or losses with other companies over time.

Invest in Black-Owned Health and Wellness Spaces: Protecting your peace can involve patronizing the practitioners at Black-owned healthcare clinics, mental health professionals, and fitness trainers/centers who understand the specific needs of the community without judgment and dismissing your voice.

Building Collaborative Networks A collective voice is more powerful than an individual one when advocating for changes in housing models and financial initiatives. The African-American Credit Union Coalition (AACUC) is a prime example of how industry professionals banded together to share information and resources to expand their own skills and use it as a pipeline for more Black representation and other resource initiatives to benefit the Black community.

Ujamaa is not just about financial independence; it is about economic justice, collective stability, and ensuring that Black communities have the resources to thrive. When Black people control their financial destiny, they can reinvest in health, education, and community well-being, leading to long-term improvements in both economic and health outcomes. As Dr. Martin Luther King Jr. once said, "We must rapidly begin the shift from a thing-oriented society to a person-oriented society." Economic empowerment must be about people first and wealth second, ensuring that financial success leads to holistic healing and sustainability.

PRINCIPLE FIVE:
NIA (PURPOSE)

Nia, meaning purpose, is the principle that emphasizes intentionality, direction, and the collective mission of uplifting the Black community. It calls for African Americans to not only live with personal purpose but to use their talents, skills, and resources to restore the dignity, culture, and health of the Black community. The pursuit of purpose is fundamentally tied to mental, emotional, and even physical well-being, as a sense of meaning in life is linked to lower stress levels, better health outcomes, and greater resilience.[259]

Historically, purpose has always been an essential force behind Black resilience and resistance. During enslavement, African Americans maintained a sense of purpose through cultural preservation, spiritual resilience, and collective survival efforts. Despite being stripped of autonomy, many found meaning in passing down oral traditions, maintaining African spiritual practices in secret, and resisting oppression in any way possible, whether through revolts, escape, or subversive acts like work slowdowns. The courageous efforts of enslaved Africans who risked their lives for liberation inspired future generations of activists, entrepreneurs, and healers to survive and thrive despite structural barriers that would attempt to block them at every turn.

Post-slavery, Black leaders and visionaries like W.E.B. Du Bois, Marcus Garvey, Mary McLeod Bethune, and Malcolm X dedicated their lives to ensuring that Black people had access to education, economic mobility, and self-determination. The Civil Rights Movement and the Black Panther Party reflected collective purpose, ensuring that healthcare, education, and social justice were prioritized for Black communities. Today, Nia is reflected in the rise of Black entrepreneurship, grassroots activism, and wellness movements focused on healing and empowering the community. However, systemic barriers continue to create obstacles, leaving many Black individuals struggling to find a sense of purpose amidst economic instability, racial discrimination, and intergenerational trauma.

Impact on Holistic Health

Mental & Emotional Health:

Studies show that individuals with a strong sense of purpose experience lower rates of depression and anxiety.[260] For African Americans, whose daily lives are often impacted by racial trauma and systemic oppression, having a clear purpose can serve as a protective factor against hopelessness and stress. Community-based purpose, such as engaging in activism or mentoring youth, fosters positive identity formation, reinforcing a sense of worth and belonging.

Physical Health:

Research indicates that a strong sense of purpose lowers mortality risk, thereby improving health and longevity throughout adulthood.[261] Black individuals who engage in purpose-driven activities, such as cultural storytelling, faith-based service, or health advocacy, often experience better health outcomes than those who feel disconnected from their cultural roots. Purpose-driven living also influences health behaviors, as people who feel their lives have meaning are more likely to prioritize self-care, proper nutrition, and regular physical activity.

Spiritual Health:

Many African spiritual traditions emphasize that every individual has a divine purpose—a calling that connects them to their ancestors, the community, and our creator. This belief provides spiritual grounding, helping Black individuals navigate racism-induced stress with a greater sense of inner strength. Faith-based institutions and community organizations often reinforce the principle of Nia by providing spaces for spiritual healing, cultural celebration, and empowerment.

Community Health:

The principle of Nia is visible in the Black educational movement, with organizations such as the Freedom Schools of the 1960s and today's Afrocentric schools, which teach Black children about self-determination, cultural history, and collective responsibility. Purpose-driven health initiatives, such as community farming projects, mental health support groups, and youth mentorship programs, actively contribute to better health and well-being for entire Black neighborhoods.

Practical Applications for Nia in Daily Life

Engage in Cultural and Historical Learning: Make it a community event to discuss great books, documentaries, and films on Black history and culture. Debate about it, laugh about it, cry about it—just do it together. Understanding Black history and heritage strengthens self-worth and communal pride and provides a sense of belonging and purpose.

Develop and Share Your Gifts: Your purpose was meant to be expressed for the benefit of others, while you enjoy the ride of expressing, so do not keep it to yourself; share it with the world. Whether through art, activism, teaching, or entrepreneurship, use your skills to contribute to the collective upliftment of the Black community and humanity at-large. Continue exploring new routes of expression until you find what aligns with your passion the most.

Mentor and Support the Next Generation: Purpose is amplified through nurturing and guiding young people. Our impact extends far beyond us and far into the future because of those seeds cultivated in the rich, receptive soil of young minds ready, willing, and eager to grow. It is the responsibility of the community to pour in the love, support, and cultural education to help them flourish in the unfoldment of their own purpose.

Prioritize Health and Wellness as a Purpose: As long as you have a pulse, you have a purpose; be intentional about keeping them both healthy. View self-care and health maintenance as acts of resistance, ensuring that future generations inherit a legacy of wellness, not just struggle.

Support Purpose-Driven Black Organizations: It is empowering to see how the community benefits from organizations and other Black-led institutions that are distributing much-needed resources and services that lessen the socioeconomic burden. Exercise your ability to pay it forward, whether through donations, volunteer work, or advocacy, however you choose to give, just give.

Nia reminds us that our lives are deeply interconnected and that true healing comes not only from personal fulfillment but also from contributing to the greater good. In a world that often attempts to devalue Black life, reclaiming purpose is a revolutionary act, one that empowers, heals, and strengthens both individuals and the community as a whole. As Maya Angelou once said, "If you're going to live, leave a legacy. Make a mark on the world that can't be erased." Let the world know you existed and that you existed well! By embracing Nia, as African Americans, we can transform generational trauma into generational purpose, ensuring that the future is one of wholeness, wellness, and empowerment.

PRINCIPLE SIX:
KUUMBA (CREATIVITY)

Kuumba, meaning creativity, is the principle that urges African Americans to use their creative gifts to uplift, heal, and transform the community. Creativity is not only about our artistic expression; it is a catalyst for resistance, survival, and healing. It manifests in music, storytelling, visual arts, activism, and even innovative problem-solving to counter systemic oppression. Throughout history, Black creativity has been a vehicle for both resistance and resilience, whether through the spirituals of the enslaved, the explosive artistic and intellectual expression of the Harlem Renaissance, or the powerful lyricism of hip-hop. Creativity has served as a form of protest, therapy, and community building, allowing African Americans to tell our stories on our own terms while reclaiming agency over our own narrative.

During slavery, African Americans were systematically denied literacy and artistic outlets, yet they created coded songs (spirituals) to communicate escape plans, designed quilts with hidden messages, and maintained African-inspired dance and drumming traditions despite punishments for doing so. This resilience through creativity is evidence of how deeply expression is tied to survival. In the 20th century, movements like the Harlem Renaissance (1920s) and the Black Arts Movement (1960s-1970s) used creativity to redefine Black identity and challenge racist narratives. Writers such as Langston Hughes, visual artists like Jacob Lawrence, and performers such as Nina Simone used their craft to reclaim Black cultural pride and resistance.

The birth of hip-hop in the Bronx in the 1970s is a leading example of Kuumba as a response to systemic oppression. Hip-hop emerged from Black communities devastated by redlining, underfunded schools, police violence, and economic disinvestment. It provided a creative outlet for young people to express their reality, using music (DJ's), dance (breakdancing), visual art (graffiti), and spoken word (rap) to articulate the struggles and aspirations of a marginalized community. The early hip-hop movement was both a survival mechanism and a form of cultural preservation, reclaiming African oral traditions and storytelling in a modern-day format. Today, although more commercialized than traditional, hip-hop remains one of the most influential art forms globally, shaping not only music but politics, fashion, and social activism.

Kuumba is also reflected in the surge of contemporary fiction trailblazed by Terry McMillan in the early 1990's that provided the literary art form of Black Love and the lived Black experience. Stories that would also be told on Black-owned creative platforms, such as Tyler Perry Studios, Issa Rae's production company, and Ava DuVernay's independent distribution company ARRAY, each ensuring that Black narratives are told through an authentic lens. Black creativity is further strengthened through Afrofuturism, which reimagines Blackness beyond oppression, merging culture with technology and speculative fiction to create new visions of possibility. Whether it is through wearing our bold colors, flexing fly hairstyles, speaking vernacular language, or striding and strutting with that Black swag, the African American community continues to find new ways of resistance and resilience through creative expression of life. The ingenuity and creativity we bring to life and culture is our own secret sauce.

Impact on Holistic Health

Mental & Emotional Health:

Creative expression is a proven method for reducing stress and trauma. Studies show that engaging in various forms of art therapy can be beneficial in lowering cortisol levels, which also contributes to a positive impact on reducing anxiety and depression.[262] There is power in creative expression, especially when shared in groups, that supports a greater sense of well-being and community cohesion. Hip-hop therapy, a mental health treatment pioneered by Social Work Clinician Edgar Tyson in 1996, is now used in clinical psychology to help Black youth process trauma, giving them a creative medium to work through pain and resilience that authentically intertwines their voice with cultural expression.

Physical Health:

Movement-based creativity, such as African dance, step, or drumming, has physical health benefits, improving cardiovascular function, flexibility, and coordination. Music in general has been shown to be very beneficial to health and well-being. In addition, various research studies also indicate that listening to Black music genres like jazz, gospel, and African drumming has a plethora of health benefits as well, that range from reduced cortisol to reduced blood pressure and lowering the risks of cognitive decline.[263]

Spiritual Health:

Many African spiritual traditions incorporate music, storytelling, and artistic rituals as essential to healing and connection with the divine. Creativity is a sacred practice that allows individuals to reclaim their ancestral power. Afrofuturism and spiritual expression in art found in works by Octavia Butler reinforce the idea that Black people are not confined by oppression but are creators of our own destiny.

Community Health:

Creativity fosters cultural continuity, ensuring that African traditions and historical narratives are preserved for future generations. Black-owned creative businesses, art therapy programs, and community arts initiatives provide spaces for healing, empowerment, and economic mobility.

Practical Applications for Kuumba in Daily Life

Engage in a Creative Practice: Whether through writing, painting, dance, spoken word, or photography, prioritize creativity within the community as a form of self-expression and communal healing. Drop in a class or two, make it a planned friends outing, or nothing beats a good ole-fashioned family talent show.

Support Black Artists and Creators: Identifying with and seeing ourselves represented in various forms of art deepens our cultural pride. We walk a bit taller, strut a bit stronger, when it is interpreted as tastefully done. Therefore, show that there is a need and appreciation by investing in Black-led films, books, galleries, and performances that tell authentic Black stories so the community as a whole can benefit.

Use Art as Activism: Painting empowering murals and writing songs of liberation and healing, it doesn't matter what type of creativity you deliver to inspire the world; it matters that you release it to circulate to your community or the masses. Follow the lead of creatives like Spike Lee, Ryan Coogler, Ta-Nehisi Coates, and Kara Walker, who use their platforms to challenge injustice and elevate Black narratives.

Incorporate African Aesthetic in Daily Life: Afrocentric fashions can be worn anytime of the year and are not just limited to Juneteenth, the week of Kwanzaa, and Black history month. Take pride in clothing made with our curvaceousness in mind. Wearing cultural clothing is another form of resisting European ideals of what is beautiful and when it is appropriate to wear it. We reserve the right to wear our heritage clothing anytime or all the time.

Encourage Artistic Expression in Youth: Creativity fosters self-confidence and cultural pride in Black children and teens. It's important to expose young people to historical Black innovators in the arts as they develop their own unique representation. The Black church has always been a place to nurture and showcase various forms of artistic expression in a supportive environment. Youth can also access local community centers, libraries, and non-profit organizations to provide platforms to introduce and enhance creative skill sets.

Kuumba reminds us that creativity is a form of power, a tool to heal, resist, and reimagine the future. Creativity allows us as African Americans to reclaim narratives, express emotions, and build strong cultural legacies, whether through art, music, storytelling, or innovation. As Chuck D of Public Enemy once said, "Rap is Black America's CNN." Original Hip-hop and other forms of Black artistic expression provides a platform to give voice to the voiceless, ensuring that the realities, dreams, and struggles of the authentic Black experience are not erased, but amplified. Through creative expression, African Americans can break generational cycles of trauma and continue to move towards healing and liberation.

PRINCIPLE SEVEN:
IMANI (FAITH)

Imani, meaning faith, calls for a deep belief in oneself, one's people, and the collective capacity to overcome oppression and create a better future. Faith has been an essential tool for survival, allowing African Americans to persist through enslavement, systemic racism, and ongoing social injustices. Faith is not just about spiritual or religious belief; it extends to trust in one's abilities, confidence in the community, and the unwavering hope that justice and liberation are possible. It is a mental, emotional, and spiritual anchor, ensuring that despite centuries of systematic attempts to break Black resilience, we have an internal power, a divine intelligence, greater than ourselves that is working in, through, and as us to ensure we continue to rise, heal, and thrive.

Throughout history, Imani has manifested in both spiritual and secular ways, providing the strength necessary to navigate adversity. During enslavement, African spiritual traditions were maintained despite forcibly converting the enslaved to Christianity. Many infused Christianity with African spiritual practices, creating what we now recognize as Black church culture. Included in this culture is theatrical sermons, call-and-response worship, soul-stirring gospel music, and deep communal support. In the periods following the Emancipation Proclamation, the Black church was a spiritual refuge and a center for tangible community life resources and self-renewal. It provided education, food, legal aid, and economic support to Black families navigating a hostile society. There was a shared faith that helped sustain the community during desolate times, reinforcing the belief that freedom and justice would one day be realized. The Black church became the foundation of resistance movements, from Booker T. Washington's Tuskegee Institute to the formation of the National Association for the Advancement of Colored People (NAACP) chapters in church basements.

Today, Imani is reflected in movements like Black Lives Matter, the rise of Afrocentric wellness initiatives, and increasing Black entrepreneurship. Theologian James Cone, in *God of the Oppressed*, reminds us that faith and liberation go hand in hand. Cone and other scholars emphasize that Black faith has always been tied to spiritual and physical freedom, demonstrating that African Americans have never accepted oppression as their fate. Spiritual and religious practices continue to serve as an anchor for the Black community, providing solace in the midst of oppressive conditions and injustice. Even amid modern-day oppression, faith sometimes feels like the last thing we have to hold on to. Faith continues to serve as a guiding force for self-determination and healing as we are reminded again and again in the foot-stomping gospel classic that "trouble don't last always."

Impact on Holistic Health

Mental & Emotional Health:

Studies show that faith-based coping strategies reduce depression, anxiety, and PTSD symptoms.[264] Having faith in one's purpose and community fosters greater resilience against the psychological toll of racism. Faith-based support groups offer emotional healing for Black people who feel isolated in predominantly white spaces.

Physical Health:

Research indicates that individuals who actively practice faith and spirituality live longer through a variety of mechanisms that include but are not limited to having a life's purpose, positive coping skills, social support, and stress reduction.[265] When faith-based communities promote healthy lifestyles, such as plant-based diets or regular fasting practices, which can also aid in metabolic regulation, it helps improve the health of the community.

Spiritual Health:

Faith allows Black people to reconnect with their ancestors and cultural roots, reinforcing a sense of purpose and belonging. Spiritual connectedness to the creator and understanding that interconnected relationship with all things was a central understanding to traditional African culture and healing practices. Interacting with life as a representative of God being a part of it all disrupts the compartmentalized paradigm dominant in western ideology. Thereby, interconnectedness fosters a greater opportunity for holistic well-being within the Black culture.

Community Health:

Faith-based institutions continue to serve as centers of Black empowerment and leadership, providing food assistance, housing support, mental health counseling, and activism where funding is available to aid the ongoing needs of this level of assistance. Churches also serve as mutual aid networks within Black communities reflecting faith in collective healing and success.

Practical Applications for Imani in Daily Life

Develop a Personal or Spiritual Practice: Whether through prayer, meditation, ancestral veneration, or self-affirmation, cultivate faith as a daily practice. This is best done upon waking to help set the tone of your day and/or right before bed, as you allow higher levels of positive thoughts and gratitude to permeate your subconscious while you sleep.

Engage in Faith-Based Community Support: Great things happen when two or more gather together, spiritual vibration is raised, souls are energized, and bodies feel recalibrated with strength. Find a Black-led religious or spiritual group or wellness circle that is suitable to you and the evolution of your spiritual growth and development.

Speak Life into the Next Generation: Proverbs 22:6 reminds us to "Train up a child in the way they should go, and when they are old, they will not depart from it." Faith is reinforced by ensuring Black children that there is a power greater than them always working for their greater good by helping them see just how valuable, capable, and powerful they truly are. Remind children of this connection daily through regular family prayer time, discussions, and communal religious/spiritual practices so that as they become older, the planted seeds will grow with them.

Trust in Collective Power: Religious/Spiritual communities develop from a shared common interest. Joining together with them as one voice can move the needle on policies that improve Black lives. You can also support other Grassroots movements that are creating positive change within Black communities.

Reclaim African-Centered Wellness: Embrace the understanding that to be created in the essence of God is to be interconnected with everything that God created. God gave us the splendor of the earth - spend time in nature, enjoying the sun, trees, and grass you stand upon barefoot. God gave us the plants and other natural elements to bring the body back in alignment—utilize herbal medicines and holistic health practices for your wellness care. God gave us sound, vibration, and connection—use your body to move to the beat of the drum, dance, laugh, love, and heal through the oneness you feel with all living things.

Imani reminds us that faith is not passive hope but active belief in transformation. It has been the foundation of Black resilience for centuries, ensuring that even in the face of systemic oppression, African Americans continue to dream, build, and heal. As the legendary Maya Angelou said, "Bringing the gifts that my ancestors gave, I am the dream and the hope of the slave. I rise, I rise, I rise." Through faith in God, faith in self, faith in the community, and faith in the future, Imani ensures that the legacy of Black perseverance and excellence endures and flourishes.

Part IV: RECLAIMING BLACK WELLNESS

The chapter "Collectivism of Wellness" reminds us that the legacy of Black resilience is not rooted in solitary achievement but in the powerful unity of our ancestors. Enslaved Black Americans, despite the dehumanization and brutality they endured, cultivated systems of support, resistance, and healing through their communal bonds. That unity was not just a means of survival; it was a form of resistance and a foundation for collective wellness. Reclaiming that tradition through the Nguzo Saba is not merely symbolic; it is a strategic and cultural reintroduction to working together for the purpose of healing, flourishing, and long-term wellness.

In the architecture of wellness, the foundation of a healthy, thriving individual cannot be fully sustained without the integrity of a strong, culturally rooted community. Identity, culture, and self-perception form the blueprint, but it is the Nguzo Saba, the seven principles of Kwanzaa, that act as the load-bearing wall, distributing the weight of life's challenges across a collective structure. Within the Black community, where the burdens of racism, economic inequity, and intergenerational trauma are heavy, embracing principles like Ujima (collective work and responsibility) and Ujamaa (cooperative economics) offers not just cultural affirmation but a necessary framework for resilience. These principles become the infrastructure that transforms isolation into empowerment and stress into shared strength. They orient the community not just toward survival, but toward sustainable well-being rooted in ancestral wisdom and cultural continuity.

Too often, wellness in the Black community has been constructed using what can be likened to curtain walls—non-structural, easily dismantled approaches that prioritize individualized self-help over communal support. Curtain walls may offer aesthetic appeal or temporary function, but they do not bear the weight of systemic oppression, nor do they provide the kind of interdependence that buffers against chronic stress, illness, and burnout. Individual efforts are more vulnerable to collapse without reinforcing shared cultural values and a unified wellness ethos. However, when load-bearing principles like the Nguzo Saba support community wellness, they become the stabilizing force that supports the individual and strengthens the whole. In this light, unification becomes more than an ideal—it becomes the architectural necessity for optimal health, regeneration, and liberation across generations.

As we move forward in exploring what it means to not only be culturally grounded but also personally well, it becomes clear that community alone is not enough. Just as a strong house requires both structural walls and personal living spaces, our wellness must also include the intentional practice of individualized habits that nourish the body, mind, and spirit. As Audre Lorde once said, "Caring for myself is not self-indulgence; it is self-preservation, and that is an act of political warfare." These are the combined practices that fortify our inner resilience.

> *"To value ourselves rightly, infinitely, released from shame and self-rejection, implies knowing that we are claimed by the totality of life. To share in a loving community and vision that magnifies our strength and banishes fear and despair, here, we find the solid ground from which justice can flow like a mighty stream. Here, we find the fire that burns away the confusion that oppression heaped upon us during our childhood weakness. Here, we can see what needs to be done and find the strength to do it. To value ourselves rightly. To love one another. This is to heal the heart of justice." ~ Victor Lewis*

Part IV: RECLAIMING BLACK WELLNESS

CHAPTER 7:
THE 12 KEY ELEMENTS OF INDIVIDUALIZED WELLNESS: TOOLS FOR BLACK HEALTH & LONGEVITY

While collective care remains the heartbeat of Black wellness, sustaining the health of the community also depends on the daily, intentional choices made by each individual. The legacy of systemic oppression has not only disrupted communal bonds but has also demanded that Black individuals navigate personal wellness in environments that are often hostile to their health. Reclaiming wellness, therefore, requires both community action and deeply personalized practices that support the unique needs of the Black body, mind, and spirit. This final chapter introduces 12 Key Elements to Reclaim Wellness, offering practical strategies designed to restore balance, strengthen resilience, and protect against the chronic diseases that disproportionately impact African Americans. As a special addition, a bonus section will focus specifically on disease prevention, highlighting proactive measures that empower individuals to safeguard their health.

These practices are more than just recommendations; they are tools to interrupt cycles of harm and rewrite the health narrative for future generations. By embracing both collective and individualized wellness, as African Americans, we reclaim the power to change the direction of our lives and the lives of those who come after us. This is how generational healing begins: when each person commits to their well-being, knowing that their health contributes to the strength, longevity, and flourishing of the entire community. Wellness, once stolen and suppressed, becomes ours to define, protect, and pass on. The Black community gets to do just that by embracing these two complementary frameworks found in the Nguzo Saba and the Twelve Key Elements: together, it is not just practice to address disease but ultimately builds a culture of health, longevity, and empowerment, one that honors ancestral wisdom, science, and holistic practices.

ELEMENT 1–BREATH:
GROUNDING IN THE PRESENT

Breath is the most fundamental element of life. It is the first action we take upon entering the world and the last before we transition. Yet, in daily life, the power of intentional breathing is often overlooked. More than just an automatic function, breath is deeply connected to our physical, mental, emotional, and spiritual well-being.

In many African and Indigenous traditions, breath is considered sacred, a force that connects the individual to the divine, to nature, and to ancestral wisdom. In the Yoruba tradition, for example, the concept of "emi" (meaning both breath and spirit) signifies that breath is more than just oxygen exchange; it is life force energy. Likewise, ancient Kemetic (Egyptian) healing practices emphasized controlled breathwork as a means to balance the body's internal energy, calm the mind, and support overall health.

Why Breath is Essential to Whole Health

Despite its automatic nature, the way we breathe affects every system in the body. It bridges the conscious and unconscious, regulating stress levels, heart rate, blood pressure, digestion, immune function, and mental clarity.

However, poor breathing habits, such as shallow chest breathing (common in high-stress environments) or chronic mouth breathing, can contribute to fatigue, anxiety, weakened immunity, and metabolic imbalances. This is particularly relevant for African Americans, who often navigate high-stress environments that contribute to dysregulated breathing patterns and related health issues.

Physiological Impact of Breath

Oxygenation & Energy Production

Proper breathing ensures that the body's cells receive adequate oxygen, which is crucial for energy production (ATP synthesis) and metabolic function.

Shallow breathing can lead to fatigue, brain fog, and decreased endurance.

Nervous System Regulation

Deep, diaphragmatic breathing activates the parasympathetic nervous system, which induces relaxation and stress reduction.

In contrast, rapid, shallow breathing keeps the body in a chronic state of fight-or-flight, increasing cortisol levels and contributing to chronic stress-related diseases.

Cardiovascular Health

Controlled breathing has been shown to lower blood pressure and heart rate, reducing the risk of hypertension, which is most prevalent with the African American population.[266]

Studies have also demonstrated that slow, deep breathing can improve heart rate variability, which is a key marker of cardiovascular resilience and stress adaptation.[267]

Respiratory Health & Disease Prevention

Asthma disproportionately affects Black Americans, who are 30% more likely to die from asthma-related complications.[268] Breath training techniques, such as Buteyko breathing, have been shown to improve lung function and reduce asthma symptoms.

Chronic exposure to air pollution in Black communities exacerbates respiratory conditions, making breath awareness and lung-strengthening exercises essential.

How Breath Connects with Health Disparities in the Black Community

- African Americans face higher exposure to environmental toxins due to racially discriminatory housing policies and industrial zoning practices.
- Urban air pollution contributes to higher rates of asthma and chronic respiratory illnesses.
- High-stress environments (workplace discrimination, financial stress, and systemic oppression) contribute to chronic

shallow breathing, stress-induced hypertension, and anxiety disorders.

The lived Black experience presents various opportunities where the knee-jerk response to having more month than money, encountering grief and trauma, feeling slighted by daily macro and microaggressions, or even locking in on the news to see if the assailant in the featured crime was a Black person, leaves us holding our breath. We also find ourselves holding our breath at the office meeting until we can exhale in a safe space that does not cost us our job or reputation. The problem is some of us find ourselves suppressing the need to exhale (figuratively) at all. Exhaling (literally) while actually focusing on the breath brings us back to center and reconnects us with our internal power that breathed the breath of life into humankind. Anchor yourself in this truth and know that it will get you through the next moment and the next moment, and the next moment after that. Breathe and remember that you have the right to feel all your feelings and allow yourself a moment to feel them. However, keep breathing, allowing it to be controlled as you remember that you do not have to stay in the heaviness of your emotions. Keep focusing on your breath until you reach a state of calm, and with more calm comes more clarity.

Holistic Strategies to Improve Breath and Respiratory Wellness

1. Diaphragmatic (Belly) Breathing

Expanding the diaphragm while inhaling allows for greater oxygen intake and activates the relaxation response.

Practice: Inhale deeply for 4 seconds through the nose, hold for 4 seconds, and exhale for 6-8 seconds through the mouth (repeat for 5-10 minutes daily).

2. Pranayama & African Ancestral Breathwork

Pranayama (yogic breath control) and Kemetic breathing techniques help improve lung capacity, mental focus, and stress regulation.

The four-part breath (square breathing) used in African healing traditions mirrors the balanced breath cycle of inhale through the nose, hold, exhale through the mouth, and hold.

3. Singing, Humming & Chanting

Engaging in rhythmic breathing practices through music, gospel singing, and drumming helps regulate breath and enhance lung function.

Studies show that humming increases nitric oxide, which can improve respiratory function and immune strength.[269]

4. Air Purification & Environmental Advocacy

Investing in air purifiers and plants (such as aloe vera and snake plants) helps improve indoor air quality.

Supporting environmental justice initiatives ensures cleaner air in Black communities.

Breath is not just a biological function but a powerful tool for healing, self-regulation, and empowerment. By incorporating intentional breath practices, African Americans can reduce stress, improve heart health, and strengthen the respiratory system, reclaiming agency over our health despite environmental and systemic challenges.

ELEMENT 2–HYDRATION:
NOURISHING THE INNER LANDSCAPE

Water is the foundation of life and vitality. Every cell, tissue, and organ in the body depends on proper hydration to function optimally. For African Americans, dehydration is an overlooked yet critical health factor that influences a wide range of conditions, from hypertension to kidney disease, obesity, and mental fatigue.

Historically, Africans deeply respected water as a sacred and life-sustaining element. In many African spiritual traditions, water was used for ritual purification, healing, and energy alignment. However, today's lack of access to clean, quality drinking water in some Black communities has turned hydration into an issue of health, justice, and survival. The Flint Water Crisis is a primary example of water contamination in a Black community that highlights the systemic neglect that continues to create barriers to adequate hydration and overall health.

Why Hydration is Essential to Whole Health

Water regulates body temperature, flushes out toxins, lubricates joints, supports digestion, and transports nutrients. Despite its importance, pure fresh water does not have the same level of popularity as flavor filled beverages like coffee, tea, soda, and juices. Making dehydration most prevalent among young children and the elderly population, therefore adding an additional burden on the Black communities where pre-existing health conditions connected to dehydration are at higher rates.

Without proper hydration:

The brain cannot function optimally, leading to fatigue, headaches, poor focus, and mood disorders.

The heart has to work harder, increasing the risk of hypertension and cardiovascular disease.

The kidneys struggle to filter toxins, raising the likelihood of chronic kidney disease, a condition disproportionately affecting African Americans.

The skin, muscles, and joints weaken, increasing inflammation and chronic pain.

For African Americans, who are already disproportionately affected by hypertension, diabetes, and kidney disease, hydration is a powerful and economically accessible tool for disease prevention.

Physiological Impact of Hydration

Brain Function & Mental Clarity

The brain is composed of about 75% water. Even mild dehydration (1-2%) can impair cognitive function, mood stability, and focus.[270]

Chronic dehydration has been linked to higher rates of depression and anxiety.

Cardiovascular Health & Blood Pressure Regulation

Dehydration thickens the blood, making the heart work harder, which increases blood pressure and stroke risk.

African American adults are 20% more likely to have a high blood pressure diagnosis, that is more advanced and develops at an earlier age compared to other racial and ethnic groups.[271] What is also alarming is that the Black population is 30% more likely to die from heart disease than white adults.[272]

Kidney Health & Chronic Disease Prevention

African Americans make up 35% of patients with kidney failure in the U.S., contributing to a surge in dialysis centers in Black communities.[273]

Drinking enough water supports kidney filtration, preventing the buildup of toxins and kidney stones.

Metabolism & Weight Management

Sugary drinks are one of the leading contributors to obesity in Black communities, where access to clean water can be limited, making hydration from healthy sources even more critical.

How Hydration Connects with Health Disparities in the Black Community

Hydration is often overlooked as a key health disparity issue in Black communities. Factors such as:

- Limited access to clean water in urban and rural Black communities due to environmental racism (e.g., Flint Water Crisis, Jackson, MS Water Crisis).
- High consumption of sugary drinks due to aggressive marketing of sodas and juices in Black communities.
- Cost of bottled water making proper hydration financially inaccessible to low-income households.
- Mistrust of tap water due to contamination concerns, leading many to opt for less healthy alternatives.
- These systemic issues make it even more important for African Americans to be intentional about hydration choices.

When we think of water as liberation, let us not forget how our enslaved ancestors followed the rivers to lead them to freedom. Traditional Black pastors used those same rivers to sanctify souls as they performed baptism by immersion. Beyond drinking, ancestral venerations, or rituals we have at our disposal multiple uses of how water can be used in our wellness journeys. Holistic health practitioners utilize a large selection of hydrotherapy techniques to introduce the therapeutic values of water in different forms. This can involve steam infused with essential oils for detoxifying and decongesting orifices like nasal passages, the vagina, or general pores on the skin. Hot and ice-cold applications, whether via immersion in a tub or locally applied, are used to reduce pain, stimulate the parasympathetic nervous system, and support the circulatory system through vasodilation (relaxing the blood vessels) and vasoconstriction (contracting the blood vessels). All of which makes water a very valuable resource, serving the cellular level of the body from both internal and external resources.

Holistic Strategies to Improve Hydration and Water Quality

1. Drink More Water, Reduce Sugary Beverages

Aim to drink half your body weight in ounces of water daily (e.g., if you weigh 160 lbs, drink 80 oz of water daily).

Cut back on sodas, sports drinks, and processed juices, which contribute to obesity and metabolic disease.

2. Infuse Water with Natural Electrolytes

Add cucumber and/or lemon to boost hydration and mineral absorption.

Coconut water is a great natural source of potassium and hydration support.

3. Use a Water Filter

If tap water is questionable, use an activated charcoal or reverse osmosis filter.

Install a water filtration system in your home for long-term sustainable access to quality water to drink, bathe, cook, and wash fresh produce with.

4. Eat Water-Rich Foods

Fruits like watermelon, oranges, cucumbers, and berries contribute to daily hydration needs.

Avoid processed foods high in sodium, which dehydrates the body.

5. Support Water Equity & Environmental Justice

Advocate for clean water policies that hold governments accountable for infrastructure failures in Black communities.

Participate in educating communities about water rights and safe drinking options.

Hydration is one of the simplest yet most powerful wellness elements that can transform health outcomes. Proper water intake supports brain function, heart health, kidney function, weight management, and disease prevention. However, for many Black communities, hydration is also an issue of systemic inequality, making it imperative to take both individual and collective action.

ELEMENT 3–NUTRITION:
RECLAIMING FOOD AS MEDICINE

Nutrition is at the core of cellular health, disease prevention, and longevity. Every meal we consume has the potential to heal or harm, influencing the body's ability to function optimally. Yet, for African Americans, historical and systemic barriers have limited access to nutrient-rich foods, contributing to higher rates of obesity, diabetes, hypertension, and cardiovascular disease.

Before the disruption of the Transatlantic Slave Trade, West African diets were naturally rich in whole, plant-based foods, lean proteins, and healthy fats. Traditional African diets, such as those from the Senegambia region, were abundant in millet, okra, black-eyed peas, leafy greens, nuts, and fish, providing a balanced source of fiber with other macro- and micronutrients. However, enslavement drastically altered Black people's relationship with food, introducing a cycle of malnutrition, food scarcity, and processed food dependency that still affects Black communities today.

Today's health disparities are not just a matter of personal choices; they are the result of systemic oppression that has shaped food availability, affordability, and quality.

Why Nutrition is Essential to Whole Health

Food is more than fuel; it is medicine, energy, and nourishment. A nutrient-dense diet supports brain function, immunity, digestion, cardiovascular health, and emotional balance. However, the lack of access to healthy foods in many Black communities means that African Americans disproportionately suffer from nutrition-related diseases.

Without proper nutrition:

The immune system weakens, increasing vulnerability to infections and chronic illnesses.

The brain lacks essential nutrients, contributing to mental fog, depression, and anxiety.

Blood sugar and insulin levels become dysregulated, increasing the risk of diabetes and obesity.

The gut microbiome is thrown off balance, leading to digestive disorders and inflammation.

For African Americans, who experience the highest rates of metabolic diseases, nutrition is one of the most powerful and accessible tools for breaking the cycle of chronic illness.

Physiological Impact of Nutrition

Blood Sugar Regulation & Diabetes Prevention

African Americans are 1.4 times more likely to be diagnosed with diabetes than whites.[274]

A diet high in fiber, lean proteins, and healthy fats slows glucose absorption, reducing insulin spikes and lowering diabetes risk.

Heart Health & Hypertension Reduction

1 in 2 Black adults has high blood pressure, which increases stroke risks. Death by stroke is 3 times greater in the Black population ages 45-54 compared to their white counterparts.[275]

Eating potassium-rich foods like bananas, avocados, and leafy greens helps support healthy blood pressure.

Reducing sodium intake, processed foods, and fried foods can decrease the risk of hypertension.

Inflammation & Chronic Disease Prevention

Chronic inflammation contributes to obesity, cancer, autoimmune diseases, and neurodegenerative conditions.

Turmeric, ginger, leafy greens, and berries are rich in anti-inflammatory compounds that can support a reduction in oxidative stress.

Gut Health & Immune Function

70% of the immune system is housed in the gut, making nutrition, digestion, and absorption critical for disease prevention.

Fermented vegetables and grains foods are naturally high in probiotics which can support gut microbiome diversity.

How Nutrition Connects with Health Disparities in the Black Community

Nutrition-related health disparities among African Americans stem from:

- **Food deserts & food swamps** - 1 out of every 5 Black households is located in a food desert, lacking in access to fresh produce, while being oversaturated with the availability of fast food and processed food.[276]
- **Economic constraints** - Fresh, whole foods cost more than processed, calorie-dense alternatives.
- **Mistrust of the medical system** - Many Black patients are not given culturally competent nutrition guidance by healthcare providers.
- **Historical trauma & survival eating patterns** - Soul food culture, while deeply rooted in tradition, has been adapted to high-fat, high-sugar, and high-sodium diets, increasing chronic disease risk.

Let's be honest and say that while navigating the hostile terrain of racism and oppression, food has definitely been central to how we cope as Black people. Food anesthetizes the stress response as we often crave releasing our anger and frustration on crunchy, fatty, and salty snacks like chips, popcorn, pretzels, and anything batter-fried. Then there are those stressors that make us yearn for soothing our feelings with a comfort that feels like a loving hug - we get that from the softness of cookies, cakes, pies, and ice cream. Food has also anchored us in how we connect as a community when we celebrate those wins in life, birthdays, holidays, or just any excuse for us to gather and have a real good time. The element of food is pivotal to the celebration and we take the taste of it very seriously. Not just any ole body can make the macaroni and cheese

Part IV: RECLAIMING BLACK WELLNESS

for the holiday meal. You know we will not even consider going to the family cookout unless a specific relative is grilling the meat because only they know how to intersect the perfection of flavor, tenderness, and moistness on the palate. We might stop by, but we will not be fixing a plate. As much as we love the culture and connecting with one another, we can no longer afford to eat like everyday is our birthday. If we want to live vibrantly till the next birthday, we must choose healthier substitutions to give us the wellness we deserve.

Holistic Strategies to Improve Nutrition in the Black Community

1. Increase Whole, Plant-Based Foods

More dark leafy greens, legumes, sweet potatoes, and whole grains improve heart health and longevity.

Reduce intake of fried foods, processed sugars, and refined carbohydrates.

Modern variations of traditional soul food meals can be adopted without the excess salt, fat, and processed sugar found in Southern cuisine adaptations.

2. Meal Prepping & Budgeting for Health

Cooking at home using whole ingredients is more cost-effective in the short & long-term than relying on fast food.

Batch cooking nutrient-dense meals reduces reliance on unhealthy takeout options.

3. Support Black Farmers & Urban Agriculture

Initiatives like Soul Fire Farm, The Black Church Food Security Network, and Black Urban Growers help increase food access in Black communities.

Growing small home gardens or community gardens can increase access to fresh produce.

4. Advocate for Policy Changes

Support policies that increase grocery store access in Black neighborhoods and limit fast food density in low-income areas.

Push for nutrition education in schools and community health programs.

Food has the power to give or take life. African Americans have been subjected to generations of nutritional oppression, but by reclaiming ancestral food traditions, prioritizing whole foods, and advocating for food justice, we can reverse the cycle of disease and redeem health and longevity.

Part IV: RECLAIMING BLACK WELLNESS

ELEMENT 4–MOVEMENT:
RECONNECTING TO STRENGTH & VITALITY

Movement is life. The human body was designed to move, stretch, run, lift, and engage in physical activity. Yet, due to historical labor exploitation, environmental barriers, and modern sedentary lifestyles, African Americans are disproportionately affected by chronic diseases linked to inactivity, such as obesity, hypertension, and Type 2 diabetes.

Historically, Africans engaged in movement as a natural part of daily life, from hunting, farming, and dancing to spiritual and communal activities. However, during enslavement, movement became a forced tool of labor and punishment. For centuries, Black people were compelled to work in grueling conditions without rest or autonomy over their bodies, which distorted the relationship with movement. After emancipation, Black workers were still forced into physically taxing jobs with little compensation, reinforcing the idea that movement was about survival, not joy, healing, or self-care.

Today, Black communities face barriers to physical activity, including neighborhood safety concerns, lack of fitness resources, and limited green spaces. Despite these challenges, movement remains one of the most practical tools for disease prevention, longevity, and mental health resilience.

Why Movement is Essential to Whole Health

Physical activity enhances cardiovascular health, mental well-being, muscular strength, and immune function. Regular movement can significantly reduce the risk of heart disease, improve mood disorders, and enhance cognitive function.[277] However, African Americans are less likely to meet the recommended levels of physical activity, contributing to higher rates of chronic illness.

Without proper movement:

The heart weakens, increasing the risk of high blood pressure, stroke, and heart disease.

Blood sugar becomes unregulated, raising the risk of Type 2 diabetes.

Mental health suffers, as physical activity is essential in reducing anxiety, depression, and PTSD symptoms.

Joint pain and mobility issues increase, leading to early-onset arthritis and chronic pain syndromes.

For Black people, whose historical and present-day experiences are filled with compounded stressors, movement is not just exercise, it is an act of healing and liberation.

Physiological Impact of Movement

Cardiovascular Health & Hypertension Prevention

Approximately 55% of the Black population in the US has a hypertension diagnosis, which is among the highest in the world according to the American Heart Association.[278]

Regular aerobic exercise (walking, dancing, jogging, biking) can reduce blood pressure and improve heart function.

Weight Management & Diabetes Prevention

Approximately 42% of Black adults are obese, which increases the risk of diabetes, inflammation, and cardiovascular disease.[279]

Strength training and resistance exercises help regulate insulin and reduce obesity-related inflammation.

Mental Health & Stress Reduction

Physical movement increases neurotransmitters dopamine and serotonin (associated with mood), reducing symptoms of depression and anxiety.

Although Black adults are more likely to report persistent symptoms of emotional distress that can include sadness, hopelessness, or feeling like everything is an effort in comparison to their white counterparts, they are less likely to receive treatment for it.[280] In addition to mental health therapy sessions, exercise is a natural antidepressant that can help regulate emotions.

Part IV: RECLAIMING BLACK WELLNESS

Joint Health & Mobility

Movement enhances bone density and reduces the risk of arthritis, which disproportionately affects Black populations.

Stretching and yoga improve flexibility, circulation, and reduce inflammation.

How Movement Connects with Health Disparities in the Black Community

Despite the benefits of movement, African Americans face several systemic barriers to exercise and physical wellness, including:

- **Neighborhood safety concerns** - Black communities often have fewer safe parks, recreational centers, and well-lit sidewalks, discouraging outdoor activity.
- **Limited access to gyms and fitness programs** - Economic disparities make gym memberships and wellness programs unaffordable for many.
- **Workplace barriers** - Black workers are disproportionately employed in jobs that do not provide opportunities for health generating movement or wellness programs.
- **Historical trauma & perception of physical labor** - After centuries of forced labor and movement as punishment, it becomes self-defeating to view exercise as an obligation rather than a form of self-care and empowerment.

There was a time when being outdoors and being physically active as a kid was a craving, an anxiousness that I would be willing to clean every room in the whole house as a reward to go outside and play with my friends. As girls, we played double dutch jump rope, hula hooping, throwing a rock on chalk outlines to hop-scotch across, or singing Ms. Mary Mack while creatively clapping and slapping with the multiple sets of hands that joined in building our precision, speed, and coordination all at the same time. Occasionally, we stopped to watch several of the boys as they played basketball, sometimes without a hoop or a court, while other guys pulled out a sheet of cardboard and a boombox to practice breakdancing. Was it exercise or just kids having fun? Definitely both. Explore and discover new ways to reawaken the child in you that is excited every day (or at least most days – wink, wink) about movement.

Holistic Strategies to Improve Movement in the Black Community

1. Incorporate Joyful Movement into Daily Life

Dancing, gardening, hiking, and playing sports can be fun ways to move without pressure.

African dance, Capoeira, line dancing, and step routines are powerful ways to reconnect with movement and culture.

2. Create Community-Based Exercise Groups

Walking or running groups in Black neighborhoods increase motivation and safety.

Community-led programs like GirlTrek, Black Men Run, and Outdoor Afro promote wellness within Black spaces.

3. Advocate for Safe & Accessible Spaces for Exercise

Fight for more investment in community parks, walking trails, and bike lanes in Black neighborhoods.

Encourage schools and workplaces to prioritize movement breaks and wellness initiatives.

4. Use Resistance Training & Strength Building

Building muscle mass helps prevent obesity, diabetes, and osteoporosis.

Incorporating simple bodyweight exercises (squats, lunges, push-ups) into daily routines makes a difference.

5. Prioritize Holistic Movement Practices

Yoga, Tai Chi, and breathwork combine physical and mental health benefits, reducing stress and tension.

Healing movements rooted in African spirituality, such as drumming and rhythm-based exercises, restore cultural connection and wellness.

Movement is a tool of empowerment and healing, not just a strategy for weight loss or fitness. Despite centuries of enduring physical exhaustion through forced labor and systemic barriers to wellness, it is critical for African Americans to reclaim movement as an intentional act of self-care and health sovereignty.

ELEMENT 5–CIRCULATION:
STIMULATING VITAL FLOW

Circulation is the foundation of vitality, ensuring that oxygen, nutrients, and immune cells reach every part of the body while removing waste and toxins. The blood, lymphatic, and cardiovascular systems all work together to keep the body nourished and free of harmful buildup. However, due to systemic health disparities, dietary patterns, and environmental stressors, African Americans face disproportionate risks of circulation-related diseases, including hypertension, heart disease, stroke, diabetes, and poor limb circulation (peripheral artery disease).

Historically, forced labor, poor nutrition, and extreme physical exertion without proper recovery took a toll on the circulatory health of enslaved Africans. The legacy of physical trauma, nutritional deprivation, and environmental toxins has continued to impact Black health outcomes, making circulatory wellness a crucial aspect of disease prevention and longevity.

Why Circulation is Essential to Whole Health

Good circulation ensures that:

Oxygen and nutrients reach tissues and organs, preventing fatigue and cell damage.

The immune system functions optimally by transporting white blood cells to fight infections.

Toxins and metabolic waste are removed efficiently, reducing inflammation and disease risk.

Brain function remains sharp, reducing the risk of cognitive decline, brain fog, and stroke.

The heart pumps blood effectively, lowering hypertension and cardiovascular disease risk.

Without healthy circulation, the risk of high blood pressure, diabetes complications, poor wound healing, and even amputation increases significantly.

Part IV: RECLAIMING BLACK WELLNESS

Physiological Impact of Circulation

Heart Health & Hypertension Prevention

African Americans develop high blood pressure at younger ages than any other group and are twice as likely to have a stroke compared to white adults.[281]

High sodium diets, stress, and lack of movement contribute to poor circulation and arterial damage.

Incorporating potassium-rich foods (bananas, leafy greens, sweet potatoes) and movement improves blood flow and reduces the risk of hypertension.

Peripheral Artery Disease (PAD) & Diabetes Complications

African Americans over 40 years of age are twice as likely to suffer from PAD, which restricts blood flow to the legs, increasing the risk of pain, infections, and amputation.[282]

Poor circulation in diabetes can lead to nerve damage (neuropathy) and slow wound healing, increasing the risk of limb loss.

Lifestyle interventions, including hydration, exercise, and plant-based foods, can significantly improve circulation and reduce complications.

Cognitive Function & Stroke Prevention

African Americans have the highest stroke rates in the U.S., with associated mortality at 3 times the rate as their white counterparts.[283]

Poor circulation reduces oxygen flow to the brain, increasing the risk of stroke, memory loss, and early dementia.

Omega-3 fatty acids, dark leafy greens, and aerobic exercise enhance brain blood flow, reducing stroke and cognitive decline.

Lymphatic System & Immune Health

The lymphatic system is a network of vessels that helps remove toxins, fight infections, and regulate fluid balance.

Unlike blood circulation, the lymphatic system has no pump—it relies on movement, deep breathing, and hydration to function properly.

Rebounding (jumping on a mini-trampoline), dry brushing, and massage therapy improve lymphatic drainage and toxin removal.

How Circulation Connects with Health Disparities in the Black Community

Despite the importance of circulation, African Americans face systemic barriers that contribute to poor cardiovascular health and circulation issues:

- **Limited access to fresh, whole foods** – Many Black communities lack grocery stores with heart-healthy options, increasing reliance on processed, high-sodium foods that elevate blood pressure.

- **Chronic stress and systemic racism** – The constant exposure to racism and discrimination increases cortisol levels, contributing to chronic inflammation and hypertension.

- **Medical bias and underdiagnosis** – Black patients are less likely to be referred for cardiovascular screenings and intervention compared to white patients, leading to delayed diagnosis and worse outcomes.[284]

- **Environmental toxins and pollution** – Black neighborhoods have higher rates of air pollution, which is directly linked to increased rates of heart disease and stroke.

To flow is a steady state of continuous natural movement. There is freedom that exists in a flow; it moves with ease and with grace as long as there are no disturbances or other external factors disrupting the flow. It will do what it was designed to do and flow where it was naturally designed to flow. In light of that, the most prevalent condition in the Black community is high blood pressure, indicating there is a disruption to the flow and circulation of our blood. Beyond the physiology of stress-provoking hypertension (discussed in Chapter 4), it is important to consider the condition metaphysically as well.

Since the time beginning with forced migration into the United

Part IV: RECLAIMING BLACK WELLNESS

States through present-day reality, Black Americans have been denied the ability to physically live and move (completely) freely in a steady, continuous, and natural state. We, as a collective body, have not been afforded that option, irrespective of wealth, fame, and fortune. As we are reminded that even reaching Black billionaire status does not offer the same protections from public crucifixion when laws have been violated. Crimes, I might add, that model legalized behaviors of and by their historical oppressors. The truth is, unresolved trauma transcends socioeconomic status as it manifests in a myriad of ways. Meanwhile, white billionaire criminals benefit from discrete exemption or management from publicized scrutiny that holds their legacy intact.

Nonetheless, the point is, there are very serious implications to being stripped of the spirituality, culture, and customs of our native land. Our ancestors were given a new understanding of God and left to build an identity through the lens of Eurocentric ideals, norms, and values for the sake of survival, all of which have disrupted everything about the natural internal and external flow of Black people. When combined with the unnatural state of dehumanization, racism, and oppression in the environment that we live in, it is insane to think that diseases of the circulatory flow would NOT manifest. Especially when you factor in the often unrecognized, unspoken, and unhealed depth of psychological trauma (discussed in Ch. 3).

Holistic Strategies to Improve Circulation in the Black Community

1. Prioritize Heart-Healthy Nutrition

Increase intake of potassium-rich foods like avocados, bananas, beans, and dark leafy greens to balance blood pressure.

Reduce processed foods, sugar, and excess sodium, which contribute to high blood pressure and arterial stiffness.

Incorporate foods high in nitric oxide (beets, garlic, pomegranates) to improve vascular health and blood flow.

2. Engage in Cardiovascular & Resistance Training

Walking, jogging, cycling, and swimming improve heart function and circulation.

Strength training (weightlifting, resistance bands) enhances blood vessel flexibility and reduces PAD risk.

Yoga and Tai Chi reduce stress while improving circulation and mobility.

3. Stay Hydrated & Use Herbal Teas for Circulation

Hydration is essential for keeping blood viscosity low and preventing clot formation.

Herbs like cayenne pepper, ginger, and turmeric support blood flow and anti-inflammation.

Drinking hibiscus tea is a natural herb that has been shown to effectively manage stage 1 hypertension.[285]

4. Reduce Stress & Practice Deep Breathing

Chronic stress constricts blood vessels, increasing hypertension risk.

Practicing deep belly breathing, meditation, and mindfulness lowers stress hormones and supports circulation.

Nature exposure and grounding (walking barefoot on the earth) help regulate the nervous system and blood flow.

5. Advocate for Environmental and Healthcare Equity

Push for policies that reduce environmental pollutants in Black communities, which directly impact heart health.

Demand fair and equal access to cardiovascular healthcare, including screenings, treatments, and preventative care.

Circulation is the foundation of vitality and longevity, yet African Americans suffer the highest rates of hypertension, stroke, and cardiovascular disease due to historical and systemic inequities. By prioritizing heart-healthy habits, movement, hydration, and stress reduction, we can improve circulation and reclaim our wellness.

ELEMENT 6–DIGESTION:
THE ROOT OF HEALTH AND DISEASE

Digestion is the gateway to overall wellness, influencing immune function, mental health, metabolism, and chronic disease prevention. The digestive system is responsible for breaking down food, absorbing nutrients, and eliminating waste, ensuring that the body receives the fuel it needs to function. For African Americans, gut health is a critical but often overlooked aspect of health disparities. Due to historical dietary shifts, food insecurity, stress, and environmental toxins, the Black community suffers from higher rates of digestive-related cancers such as colorectal and pancreatic cancer.[286]

Historically, prior to captivity, Africans maintained a plant-based, fiber-rich diet, but during enslavement, their diets became limited to nutrient-deficient foods like cornmeal and pork scraps. This dietary deprivation laid the foundation for generational health issues that continue to impact the Black population today.

Why Digestion is Essential to Whole Health

Healthy digestion ensures:

Efficient absorption of essential nutrients, preventing deficiencies that contribute to disease.

A balanced gut microbiome, which supports immune function, mental health, and metabolic regulation.

Elimination of toxins, reducing the risk of inflammation and chronic illness.

Regulation of blood sugar and weight, helping to prevent obesity and diabetes.

A strong connection between gut health and mental health, as the gut produces over 90% of the body's serotonin (the "feel-good" neurotransmitter).

Without proper digestion, individuals are at risk of malnutrition, immune dysfunction, inflammation, and mental distress.

Physiological Impact of Digestion

Colorectal Cancer & Digestive Cancers

African Americans are 20% more likely to be diagnosed with colorectal cancer in the US and a 40% increased mortality rate compared to the white population.[287]

Low fiber intake, high-fat diets, and inadequate screenings contribute to late-stage diagnoses.

Cruciferous vegetables, fermented foods, and high-fiber diets significantly reduce risk.

Gastroesophageal Reflux Disease (GERD) & Heartburn

Black individuals have a high prevalence of GERD, which can increase the risk of esophageal cancer.

High-fat diets, processed foods, and stress weaken the lower esophageal sphincter, leading to acid reflux.

Eating smaller meals, avoiding acidic foods, and consuming alkaline-rich foods help manage GERD naturally.

Gut Dysbiosis & Microbiome Imbalance

The gut microbiome is a collection of trillions of bacteria that influence digestion, immunity, and mental health.

Diets high in processed foods and low in fiber destroy beneficial gut bacteria, leading to inflammation.

Fermented foods (kimchi, sauerkraut, yogurt) and prebiotics (onions, garlic, asparagus) support a healthy microbiome.

Diabetes, Insulin Resistance, & Blood Sugar Regulation

African Americans are 1.4 times more likely than whites to be diagnosed with diabetes, largely due to processed food consumption, sugar intake, and high-carb diets.[288]

Fiber slows glucose absorption, preventing insulin spikes and reducing diabetes risk.

Whole grains, legumes, and plant-based proteins improve insulin sensitivity.

The Gut-Brain Connection & Mental Health

The gut produces neurotransmitters like serotonin and dopamine, which regulate mood.

Poor digestion and inflammation are linked to anxiety, depression, and cognitive decline.

A healthy gut reduces stress, improves sleep, and enhances emotional resilience.

How Digestion Connects with Health Disparities in the Black Community

- **Food Deserts & Limited Access to Nutrient-Dense Foods** Black communities are disproportionately located in food deserts, where fresh produce is scarce. The reliance on fast food and processed meals increases the risk of poor digestion, obesity, and diabetes.

- **High Consumption of Processed & Fried Foods**—Southern-style diets high in fried foods, sugar, and refined carbs increase inflammation and digestive disorders. Shifting to fiber-rich, plant-based meals improves gut health and prevents chronic disease.

- **Medical Racism in Digestive Health Treatment**—Black patients are less likely to receive colonoscopies, GERD treatments, and digestive health screenings. Implicit bias in medical settings delays proper diagnoses and life-saving interventions.

- **Historical Dietary Shifts & Generational Impact** - The transition from African plant-based diets to Westernized high-fat, low-fiber diets contributed to long-term digestive issues. Reclaiming ancestral eating patterns can help restore gut health and overall well-being.

At the core of Naturopathic medicine is toning and optimizing gut function. An overwhelming majority of patients that I have worked with over the past decade have had some level of gastrointestinal issues. However, it is a much smaller percentage that has sought after my care specifically for those concerns because they are usually motivated by what they perceive to be more severe health conditions. Because digestion, absorption, and elimination are fundamental to properly resourcing what is needed and discarding from the body what is not, optimizing gut function significantly improves the experience of overall health and well-being. I am often told, "I thought it was just gas and bloating" or "I have always only eliminated every other day; I thought it was normal for my body." I have witnessed moods improve and patients become more motivated about life, energy enhanced for them to stick to an exercise plan, and more confidence because their skin has cleared up. Let's just say while working holistically with me, my patients have experienced more side bonuses than side effects while improving their presenting condition.

Holistic Strategies to Improve Digestion in the Black Community

1. Increase Fiber Intake

Fiber promotes regular bowel movements, gut microbiome balance, and reduced inflammation.

Consume leafy greens, whole grains, lentils, and fresh fruits daily.

2. Incorporate Fermented & Probiotic Foods

Fermented foods introduce good bacteria into the gut, reducing bloating and inflammation.

Eat kimchi, sauerkraut, and miso regularly.

3. Reduce Processed & Fried Foods

Avoid fried foods, sugary snacks, and white flour-based products, which cause gut inflammation and insulin resistance.

Opt for baked, grilled, or raw plant meals to improve digestion.

4. Drink Plenty of Water & Herbal Teas

Dehydration slows digestion and contributes to constipation.

Herbal teas like ginger, peppermint, and fennel soothe digestion and reduce bloating.

5. Manage Stress & Support the Gut-Brain Axis

Chronic stress disrupts digestion by increasing cortisol levels.

Deep breathing, meditation, and mindful eating improve gut function and reduce stress-related symptoms.

6. Prioritize Digestive Health Screenings

Colonoscopies and digestive health screenings are essential for early detection of disease.

Advocate for equal access to preventive care and nutrition education.

Digestive health is the foundation of disease prevention, mental clarity, and overall wellness. Despite systemic barriers, Black communities can reclaim their health through dietary shifts, gut-friendly habits, and access to proper care.

ELEMENT 7–DETOXIFICATION:
CLEANSING TOXINS AS A LIFESTYLE

Detoxification is the body's natural process of eliminating toxins, allowing cells to function optimally and preventing disease. The digestive tract, liver, kidneys, skin, lungs, and lymphatic system work together to remove metabolic waste, environmental pollutants, and harmful substances that accumulate over time.

For African Americans, detoxification is particularly critical due to higher exposure to environmental toxins, poor air quality, contaminated water sources, and processed food consumption. Research shows that Black communities are disproportionately affected by pollutants from industrial plants, chemical runoff, and food additives, all of which contribute to increased rates of chronic illness, autoimmune disorders, and cancer.[289]

Historically, West African cultures utilized plant-based, whole-food diets rich in cleansing herbs, bitter greens, and detoxifying practices like fasting and herbal tonics. However, the dietary shifts caused by slavery, economic oppression, and food insecurity introduced toxins into Black communities that have been challenging to remove.

Why Detoxification is Essential to Whole Health

A properly functioning detoxification system:

Prevents the accumulation of harmful toxins that contribute to disease.

Supports liver health, reducing the risk of fatty liver disease and metabolic dysfunction.

Enhances skin clarity, energy levels, and digestion.

Boosts immunity, reducing the likelihood of chronic inflammation and infections.

Eliminates excess hormones that contribute to hormonal imbalances and reproductive disorders.

Without effective detoxification, toxins build up in the body, leading to fatigue, brain fog, digestive issues, skin problems, weight gain, and a weakened immune system.

Physiological Impact of Detoxification

Liver Function & Toxin Elimination

The liver is a primary detox organ in the body, breaking down toxins and eliminating them through bile and urine.

High-fat diets, alcohol consumption, and environmental toxins can overload the liver, leading to non-alcoholic fatty liver disease (NAFLD).

Foods like dark leafy greens, beets, turmeric, cruciferous vegetables, and dandelion root tea support liver detoxification.

Kidney Function & Hydration

The kidneys filter out toxins from the blood, but dehydration and high-sodium diets can impair function.

African Americans have the highest rates of kidney disease compared to other racial and ethnic groups, making up more than 35% of dialysis patients despite being only 13.5% of the U.S. population.[290]

Hydration, herbal teas, and avoiding processed foods help maintain kidney health.

Lymphatic System & Immune Health

The lymphatic system removes waste, carries immune cells, and prevents infections.

Unlike blood circulation, the lymphatic system lacks a pump, meaning movement is necessary for detoxification.

Rebounding, dry brushing, and lymphatic massage improve drainage and toxin removal.

Heavy Metal & Environmental Toxin Exposure

Black communities face higher exposure to lead, mercury, and industrial toxins due to environmental racism.

The Flint Water Crisis exposed thousands of Black families to toxic lead levels, increasing the risk of neurological damage, kidney failure, and developmental disorders.[291]

Cilantro, chlorella, and spirulina help remove heavy metals from the body.

How Detoxification Connects with Health Disparities in the Black Community

- **Food Contamination & Processed Foods** - Black communities experience higher exposure to food additives, dyes, and preservatives, which increase the risk of metabolic disorders. Organic, whole foods help reduce the toxin burden on the body.

- **Air & Water Pollution in Black Neighborhoods** - Studies show that predominantly Black communities have higher levels of industrial pollution, leading to respiratory diseases and cancer. Environmental toxins contribute to asthma, eczema, and autoimmune disorders.

- **Lack of Access to Detoxifying Foods & Supplements** - Many Black neighborhoods lack access to fresh, organic foods, making it harder to reduce toxin exposure. Incorporating detoxifying herbs and whole foods can help counteract the effects of environmental toxins.

- **Chemical Straighteners & Black Women** - Studies show that Black women are at an increased risk for uterine cancer and fibroid tumors associated with frequency and long-term use of chemical hair straightening products.

Toxins! Everywhere all at once. Just because we cannot see them does not mean they are not present. It is important to know that they create excessive damage when we allow them to accumulate more rapidly than we are eliminating them. Unfortunately, the general population is typically not intentional about stopping and paying attention long enough to give the body a toxic break. This was not the case for one reader who independently completed the liquid fasting detoxification protocol and supplemental therapies outlined in my book *Detox-Style* and later became a patient. I was informed of how it helped yield incredible results of a full-body reset. The patient witnessed their body expelling an abundance of toxins from multiple orifices as the body was allowed ten days of uninterrupted time to eliminate and cleanse without the distraction of digesting food. I was told how profound the experience was for the patient, not just during the actual detox but more significantly afterwards. Not only was the patient feeling new and improved, but they also gained more insight into personal health, and they noticed how their body responded when simple foods were slowly reintroduced, particularly those that triggered disturbances. The patient independently accomplished a level of success towards improved wellness that later served as a launching pad for our more in-depth personalized wellness sessions.

Holistic Strategies to Support Detoxification in the Black Community

1. Increase Hydration & Herbal Teas

Drink at least half your body weight in ounces of water daily to flush toxins from the liver and kidneys.

Herbal teas like burdock root, dandelion leaf, and nettle cleanse the bloodstream and support detoxification.

2. Consume Detoxifying Foods

Cruciferous vegetables (broccoli, kale, cabbage) support liver detox pathways.

Beets, lemon water, and garlic help eliminate toxins from the bloodstream.

3. Engage in Movement & Sweating

Exercise increases circulation, improving lymphatic drainage and toxin removal.

Sweating through sauna use, hot yoga, or cardio helps eliminate heavy metals.

4. Reduce Processed Foods & Environmental Toxins

Eliminate processed meats, artificial sweeteners, and chemical-laden personal care products.

Opt for natural household cleaners and non-toxic beauty products.

5. Incorporate Fasting & Intermittent Fasting

Periodic fasting gives the body time to detoxify, reducing inflammation and oxidative stress.

Water fasting improves glucose dysregulation and promotes cellular repair.

Detoxification is a fundamental aspect of wellness, particularly for African Americans who face increased exposure to environmental toxins and processed foods. By incorporating detoxifying foods, hydration, movement, and environmental awareness, we can reduce our toxin burden and promote long-term health. More info on how to regularly detox for improved health can be found in my book *Detox-Style: Creating a Healthy Lifestyle Through Daily Holistic Detoxification Practices*.[292]

Part IV: RECLAIMING BLACK WELLNESS

ELEMENT 8 – REST:
SACRED STILLNESS AND RENEWAL

Rest is another overlooked yet essential component of holistic wellness. It is the time when the body repairs, the mind resets, and the spirit rejuvenates. Without adequate rest, every other wellness element, including digestion, detoxification, immunity, and mental clarity begins to decline.

For African Americans, chronic sleep deprivation and inadequate rest have been deeply ingrained through both historical and contemporary systemic oppression. Enslaved Africans were forced into backbreaking labor from sunup to sundown, often with little sleep or time for a full recovery. Even after emancipation, the legacy of economic exploitation meant that Black workers had to work longer hours in low-paying jobs, often sacrificing sleep to survive.

Today, these patterns continue. African Americans are more likely to experience sleep deprivation due to economic stress, environmental factors, shift work, and racialized stressors.[293] The inability to rest, restore, and recover has far-reaching effects on cardiovascular health, immune function, mental well-being, and longevity.

Why Rest is Essential to Whole Health

Regenerates the body, repairing cells and restoring energy.

Strengthens the immune system, reducing susceptibility to infections.

Balances hormones, regulating metabolism, stress response, and reproductive health.

Improves mental clarity and emotional resilience.

Reduces inflammation and the risk of chronic diseases.

When sleep and rest are compromised, the body experiences chronic stress, hormonal imbalances, and increased risk of disease.

Physiological Impact of Rest and Sleep

Sleep and Cardiovascular Health

Sleep deprivation raises blood pressure and increases the risk of heart disease.

African Americans have the highest rates of hypertension, at 44% in comparison to whites. In addition they have greater occurrences of inadequate rest due to shorter sleep and sleep disturbances, which are major contributing factors to high blood pressure.[294]

Deep sleep reduces stress hormones and allows blood vessels to relax.

Sleep and Metabolism

Insufficient sleep is linked to obesity, diabetes, and metabolic syndrome.

Studies show that poor sleep quality is associated with a higher risk of insulin resistance and weight gain, both of which are more prevalent in Black communities.[295]

Sleep helps regulate appetite hormones like leptin and ghrelin, reducing cravings for unhealthy foods.

The Role of Rest in Mental and Emotional Health

Lack of sleep increases cortisol (stress hormone) levels, contributing to anxiety and depression.

Studies show that Black Americans experience higher rates of race-related socioeconomic factors that lead to disturbed sleep patterns.[296]

Rest is essential for cognitive function, decision-making, and emotional balance.

How Rest Connects with Health Disparities in the Black Community

- **Racial Disparities in Sleep Disorders** - The Jackson Heart Study revealed 24% of African Americans had moderate to severe sleep apnea, but only 5% had been diagnosed by a doctor.[297] Medical racism plays a role in underdiagnosis and inadequate sleep disorder treatments.

- **Economic and Environmental Barriers to Quality Rest -** Black workers are more likely to have multiple jobs, irregular shifts, or night shifts, making consistent sleep patterns difficult. Lower-income Black neighborhoods often experience more environmental disruptions (e.g., noise, light pollution, lack of safety), affecting sleep quality.

- **Generational Trauma and Hypervigilance -** Chronic stress from racism leads to hypervigilance, where the nervous system remains in a heightened state of alertness. This hypervigilance results in sleep disturbances, difficulty relaxing, and long-term health consequences.

We can no longer afford to be about that on-the-grind life that so many of us have spoken so proudly of, including me. I know first-hand what it is like to work through the night, get off and drive straight to the next job with maybe 30-45 minutes in the parking lot to close my eyes, but too scared to because I may not wake up. The grind is real, the need for additional cash is real. Sometimes it can be controlled by adjusting other factors and sometimes it takes a minute, a long minute. In the meantime, we must become motivated to change as many elements as we can to resist the tug that "grind" has on us while it encroaches on our health and quality of life. Tricia Hersey reminds us in Rest Is Resistance: A Manifesto that, "You were not just born to center your entire existence on work and labor. You were born to heal, to grow, to be of service to yourself and community to practice, to experiment, to create, to have space, to dream, and to connect." Admit it, life is best enjoyed when we feel fully rested.

Holistic Strategies to Improve Rest in the Black Community

1. Prioritize Sleep Hygiene

Create a bedtime routine with dim lighting, relaxation techniques, and electronic-free time before sleep.

Go to bed at the same time each night to regulate the body's internal clock.

2. Improve Sleep Environment

Use blackout curtains and white noise machines to eliminate environmental disruptions.

Invest in a quality mattress and pillows to support spinal alignment and deep sleep.

3. Incorporate Stress-Reducing Practices

Meditation, deep breathing, and journaling help calm the mind before bed.

Eliminating caffeine and sugar intake in the evening hours reduces sleep disturbances.

4. Address Sleep Disorders and Seek Medical Advocacy

Black Americans are often underdiagnosed for sleep disorders like sleep apnea—advocate for proper screening and treatment.

Herbal remedies like valerian root, chamomile, and magnesium can support natural sleep regulation.

5. Practice Rest Beyond Sleep

Rest is more than just sleep, taking moments to pause, reflect, and reset throughout the day is essential.

Engage in activities that restore mental and emotional well-being, such as prayer, music, creative arts, and time in nature.

Rest is not a luxury, it is a necessity for survival and longevity. African Americans face systemic barriers to quality sleep and rest, yet by prioritizing sleep hygiene, stress management, and advocating for proper treatment, we can reclaim rest as an essential pillar of health.

ELEMENT 9 – INFLAMMATION REGULATION: REDUCING THE BODY'S ALARM SYSTEM

Inflammation is a natural immune response that helps the body fight infections and heal injuries. However, when inflammation becomes chronic, it can silently damage tissues, weaken the immune system, and contribute to nearly every major chronic disease. For African Americans, systemic inflammation is a root cause of disproportionate rates of hypertension, diabetes, heart disease, autoimmune disorders, and even cancer.[298] Many of these inflammatory conditions are linked to stress, diet, environmental toxins, and racial health disparities that expose Black individuals to a greater inflammatory burden over their lifetimes.

Historically, African healing traditions focused on anti-inflammatory nutrition and herbal medicine, which supported longevity and vitality. However, through forced dietary shifts during slavery and the introduction of processed Western foods, the Black community was systematically distanced from these healing practices, leading to an increase in inflammation-related diseases.

Why Inflammation Regulation is Essential to Whole Health

Prevents chronic diseases like diabetes, heart disease, and cancer.

Reduces joint pain, arthritis, and neurodegenerative diseases.

Strengthens the immune system and protects against infections.

Balances mental health by reducing the impact of stress hormones.

Promotes healthy aging and longevity.

Without inflammation regulation, the body remains in a constant state of stress, leading to premature aging, weakened immunity, and increased disease risk.

Physiological Impact of Chronic Inflammation

Heart Disease & Hypertension

Cardiovascular Disease is the leading cause of death, with African Americans leading in mortality rates.[299]

Chronic inflammation damages blood vessels, raises blood pressure, and increases the risk of heart attacks and strokes.

Anti-inflammatory diets rich in omega-3s, fiber, and antioxidants reduce cardiovascular inflammation.

Diabetes & Insulin Resistance

Higher obesity rates among African Americans predispose them to Type II Diabetes at twice the rate, with chronic inflammation impairing insulin function.[300]

High sugar and processed food intake increase inflammation and disrupt blood sugar regulation.

Turmeric, cinnamon, and green tea help support inflammatory markers and insulin sensitivity.

Autoimmune Disorders & Chronic Pain

Black women have the highest disease prevalence of Systemic Lupus Erythematosus, an inflammatory condition, one study shows how racial discrimination increased these patients' inflammation markers.[301]

Eliminating inflammatory foods and increasing gut health support reduces autoimmune flare-ups.

Meditation, deep breathing, and stress reduction lower inflammatory cytokines in the body.

Cancer & Cellular Damage

Chronic inflammation increases the risk of aggressive cancers, including prostate, breast, and colorectal cancer, all of which disproportionately impact Black communities.[302]

Consuming cruciferous vegetables (broccoli, kale, cabbage) and antioxidant-rich foods (berries, turmeric, green tea) protects against inflammation-induced DNA damage.

The Link Between Stress & Inflammation

Chronic racial stress increases cortisol levels, which fuels inflammation.

Stress also weakens the gut microbiome, making inflammation worse.

Mindfulness, movement, and herbal adaptogens (ashwagandha, rhodiola) helps the body modulate the stress-response.

How Inflammation Connects with Health Disparities in the Black Community

- **High-Stress Environments & Systemic Oppression -** Chronic stress from racism, economic instability, and discrimination triggers inflammatory responses that increase disease risk.
- **Processed & Inflammatory Diets -** Food deserts and financial barriers limit access to fresh, anti-inflammatory foods, increasing reliance on processed and high-sugar diets.
- **Environmental Toxins & Pollution -** Black communities experience higher exposure to air pollutants, heavy metals, and industrial toxins, all of which contribute to inflammation.
- **Medical Racism in Diagnosis & Treatment -** Black individuals are less likely to be tested for inflammatory markers and are often dismissed when reporting symptoms of chronic pain.

Walking down the driveway to the mailbox and back was manageable on a good day, but even on the very best of days, the thought of walking down the first couple of aisles of Walmart would be emotionally daunting. Patient X had to mentally prepare herself to endure the pain and exhaustion she felt while picking up a few items of groceries and personal supplies. Her body was filled with inflammation and a very long list of symptoms attached to various diseases diagnosed by her primary care physician. She could not afford holistic help, but she knew a new set of resources beyond the care she had received thus far, was imperative to her quality of life. I did not perform any magic tricks on her but after battling with debilitating pain for years, she was equally amazed as if I did. Over the next several months, as we continued to work together to minimize her systemic inflammation, she reached a point in her improvement where she was walking with no assistance, no pain, or fatigue, all around Walmart, no longer limited to the first couple of aisles. Excessive inflammation will not only inflame your body but also incapacitate it to the point that your life feels inflamed.

Holistic Strategies to Reduce Inflammation in the Black Community

1. Adopt an Anti-Inflammatory Diet

Increase intake of leafy greens, berries, fatty fish, nuts, and turmeric.

Reduce processed foods, refined sugars, and fried foods that fuel inflammation.

2. Manage Stress & Cortisol Levels

Incorporate deep breathing, yoga, and mindfulness to lower inflammation-related stress.

Engage in community healing spaces, including group therapy and support networks.

3. Hydration & Herbal Remedies

Drink plenty of water to flush out inflammatory toxins.

Herbs like ginger, turmeric, and green tea support anti-inflammation naturally.

4. Move Daily & Engage in Gentle Exercise

Regular movement reduces inflammatory cytokines and improves circulation.

Walking, stretching, and tai chi lower systemic inflammation without stressing the body.

5. Prioritize Gut Health

Consume prebiotic and probiotic foods (fermented vegetables, yogurt, kefir) to strengthen the gut microbiome.

Gut-friendly diets reduce systemic inflammation and support long-term health.

Inflammation is one of the most powerful contributors to racial health disparities. By actively reducing stress, improving diet, and using natural anti-inflammatory strategies, Black communities can regain control over our health and lower the burden of disease.

ELEMENT 10 – IMMUNE SYSTEM PROTECTION:
STRENGTHENING THE BODY'S DEFENSE

The immune system is the body's natural defense against infections, diseases, and harmful invaders. A strong immune system is essential for preventing illness, reducing the severity of diseases, and promoting longevity. However, historical and contemporary health disparities have left Black communities vulnerable to weakened immune function, increasing the risk of chronic illnesses, autoimmune disorders, and infectious diseases like COVID-19 and the flu.

Historically, enslaved Africans relied on herbal medicine, nutrient-rich diets, and communal healing practices to maintain immune resilience. However, due to generations of systemic oppression, food insecurity, environmental toxins, and medical neglect, many African Americans today face higher exposure to immune-suppressing factors, including chronic stress, poor diet, and inadequate healthcare access. Strengthening immune system protection is essential to breaking the cycle of health inequities, allowing Black individuals to thrive rather than simply survive.

Why Immune System Protection is Essential to Whole Health

Defends against viruses, bacteria, and infections.

Prevents autoimmune disorders and chronic inflammation.

Supports faster recovery from illness and injury.

Regulates stress hormones that weaken immunity.

Lowers the risk of cancer, diabetes, and cardiovascular disease.

Without a strong immune system, the body becomes more susceptible to disease, inflammation, and long-term health complications.

Physiological Impact of a Weakened Immune System

Increased Susceptibility to Infections

African Americans experienced disproportionately high mortality rates during the COVID-19 pandemic due to weakened immune responses exacerbated by systemic health disparities.[303]

Chronic stress, food insecurity, and environmental toxins contribute to immune suppression.

Higher Rates of Autoimmune Disorders

Black women are disproportionately affected by lupus, multiple sclerosis, and rheumatoid arthritis with progressively worse health outcomes, all of which are linked to immune system dysfunction.[304]

Nutrient deficiencies and chronic inflammation play a key role in autoimmune diseases.

Weakened Immunity from Chronic Stress & Racism

Studies show that the stress of racism and discrimination weakens the immune system by increasing cortisol and inflammatory cytokines.[305]

This leads to higher rates of disease susceptibility and longer recovery times from illness.

Impact of Poor Diet & Environmental Toxins

A lack of access to fresh, nutrient-dense foods deprives the immune system of essential vitamins and minerals.

Black communities are disproportionately exposed to air pollutants and industrial toxins that weaken immune function.

How Immune Health Connects with Health Disparities in the Black Community

- **Higher Rates of Infectious Disease Mortality** - Black Americans have higher death rates from pneumonia, sepsis, and other infections due to immune suppression and healthcare disparities.[306]

- **Delayed Diagnoses & Medical Mistrust**—Black individuals are less likely to receive early treatment for immune-related conditions due to medical mistrust.[307]
- **Chronic Vitamin D Deficiency**—Due to higher melanin concentration, Black individuals naturally produce less vitamin D, which is essential for immune regulation. Vitamin D deficiency is linked to higher rates of respiratory infections and autoimmune diseases.[308] Among Black women, it has also been linked to an increased risk of uterine fibroids, a condition most prevalent in this population.[309]

"Stay ready, to be ready" is a term many are familiar with, reminding us to be prepared at all times. It is safe to say COVID-19 caught the Black community off guard and became a wake-up call for the nation as the death tolls kept rising and African Americans were leading in every age group from the babies to the elders. The spotlight brought much needed, long overdue attention to the severity of the health problems that run rampant in our community. Conditions that had been normalized by the healthcare industry and many Black people, both in part built off of preexisting narratives addressed in this book (see Chapter 1). It is easier to accept conditions and not challenge their frequency when narratives of biological inferiority are held in place. Also, being consumed with day-to-day survival and all of its associated stressors, disease can easily become normalized when you personally know at least five people with hypertension and/or diabetes.

COVID-19 pulled the shower curtain back, nonetheless and exposed just how fragile the Black body was to one more condition. Becoming infected with the virus was the last straw for many before death compounded onto cells that were so compromised that there was no more fight left in them to be had. Body after body succumbed, and death rates escalated, reminding us all that there is nothing normal about having a disease diagnosis. We must maintain immune cell strength while there is nothing to fight so that when invaders come our way, the body is conditioned to demolish them on site, no questions asked.

Holistic Strategies to Strengthen the Immune System in the Black Community

1. Increase Nutrient-Dense Foods

Consume a diet rich in vitamin C, zinc, and antioxidants to support immunity.

Dark leafy greens, citrus fruits, ginger, and garlic are powerful immune boosters.

2. Manage Stress & Cortisol Levels

Chronic stress weakens immunity, making stress reduction essential.

Deep breathing, meditation, and community support reduce stress-related immune suppression.

3. Prioritize Gut Health

70% of the immune system is in the gut—probiotics and fiber-rich foods improve immune resilience.

Fermented foods like sauerkraut, tempeh, and kimchi support gut-immune health.

4. Improve Sleep & Rest

Sleep deprivation suppresses immune function—aim for at least 7-9 hours of quality sleep.

Melatonin (a hormone that regulates sleep) also plays a role in immune system repair.

5. Reduce Environmental Toxin Exposure

Limit exposure to processed foods, air pollution, and household chemicals that weaken immunity.

Use natural cleaning products and air purifiers to reduce toxic burdens.

A strong immune system is essential for preventing disease and overcoming health disparities in the Black community. By prioritizing nutrient-dense foods, stress management, gut health, and environmental awareness, we can fortify the body's natural defenses and promote longevity.

Part IV: RECLAIMING BLACK WELLNESS

ELEMENT 11 – STRESS MANAGEMENT:
CULTIVATING CALM IN A CHAOTIC WORLD

Stress is a normal part of life, but chronic, unrelenting stress is detrimental to overall health (as discussed in Chapter 4). It has been well-documented that African Americans experience higher levels of cumulative stress due to systemic oppression, economic instability, discrimination, and racialized trauma.[310] This prolonged exposure to stress leads to higher rates of hypertension, cardiovascular disease, mental health disorders, and immune dysfunction.

For centuries, stress has been a defining feature of the Black experience in America. From the trauma of enslavement to the ongoing realities of economic hardship, racial profiling, and workplace discrimination, Black individuals have been forced to navigate a world that often undermines our well-being. Yet, despite these barriers, resilience has remained a hallmark of survival. However, resilience alone is not enough. Active stress management is necessary to reduce the physical and psychological toll of chronic stress, enhance emotional well-being, and improve health outcomes.

Why Stress Management is Essential to Whole Health

Lowers the risk of heart disease, hypertension, and stroke.

Reduces chronic inflammation and supports immune function.

Improves mental health and reduces anxiety and depression.

Enhances focus, memory, and cognitive function.

Promotes emotional resilience and spiritual grounding.

Without effective stress management, the body remains in a constant state of fight-or-flight, leading to hormonal imbalances, chronic illness, and premature aging.

Physiological Impact of Chronic Stress

The Role of Cortisol in Stress and Disease

Cortisol is the body's primary stress hormone. When elevated for prolonged periods, it increases inflammation and weakens immune function.

African Americans have been found to have higher exposure to racial stress and discrimination, which can trigger higher cortisol levels, thereby increasing their risk of chronic disease.[311]

Chronic Stress and Hypertension

African Americans have the highest rates of hypertension in the world, which can be attributed to increased risk due to chronic perceived stress exposure.[312]

Chronic stress perpetually activates the sympathetic nervous system, leading to a risk of high blood pressure.

The Connection Between Stress and Mental Health Disparities

Although African Americans experience higher rates of depression and anxiety, they are less likely to receive treatment due to stigma, medical mistrust, and lack of access to culturally competent care.

Mindfulness, therapy, and community healing practices help mitigate the effects of stress on mental health.

Stress, Inflammation, and Immune Suppression

Chronic stress increases inflammatory cytokines, contributing to diseases like diabetes, cancer, and autoimmune disorders.[313]

Growing research studies indicate that stress reduction practices can lower inflammation markers, which supports overall health and well-being.[314]

How Stress Disproportionately Affects the Black Community

- **Racial Trauma and Daily Discrimination** - Racial stressors, such as structural inequities, microaggressions, workplace bias, and police brutality, contribute to long-term stress responses. The concept of 'weathering,' (discussed in Chapter 4) highlights how chronic stress accelerates aging and increases disease risk in African Americans.
- **Economic and Job-Related Stress** - Financial instability, job discrimination, and wage disparities create added stress

burdens in Black communities. Economic stress has been linked to higher rates of mental health disorders and physical illness.

- **Historical Trauma and Generational Stress -** Research on epigenetics (Discussed in Chapter 5) shows that historical trauma can alter stress responses in future generations. The impact of slavery, segregation, and racial violence is still biologically and psychologically present in Black communities today.

Walking 5 miles per day a few times a week, being intentional about making healthy food choices, taking supplements, and having a daughter as a naturopathic doctor simply was not enough to save my mother from the cumulative impact of stress. For decades, I served as her sounding board and source of comfort as she navigated the challenging terrain of workplace dissatisfaction, her discomfort perhaps not at the threshold that could have motivated her to seriously seek out employment elsewhere. Familiarity and perceived job security are reasonable desires to have at any place of employment. Although staying put sometimes comes at a higher cost than the body can afford, it sometimes comes due all at once.

My mother practiced healthier habits than most and appeared a lot healthier than most. Approximately eighteen months after retiring, she was diagnosed with cancer; this time it was in the lungs and not the breast tissue where it originally appeared 30 years earlier. She had never smoked a day in her life, yet the cumulative toll of internalized stress banged loudly on the door, startling everyone. Yelling, "It is time for you to pay up." Eighteen months later, she transitioned. Physiologically, she died from a pulmonary embolism (blood clot in the lung), but as a naturopathic doctor, who was not only her daughter but also her close confidant, I am more than aware of the burden of a lifetime of stressors that she endured. Sometimes we can practice all the right habits and it still not be enough. Believe me when I say, unmitigated stress can evolve into a hell of a debt to pay, especially for those directly involved, but also the grieving loved ones they leave behind.

Holistic Strategies to Manage Stress in the Black Community

1. Mindfulness and Meditation Practices

Mindfulness meditation has been shown to lower cortisol levels and improve emotional regulation.[315]

Practices like yoga, breathwork, and visualization can also provide daily stress relief.

2. Building Community and Support Networks

Connecting with trusted family, friends, and support groups provides emotional strength and a sense of belonging.

Faith-based and spiritual practices, historically a pillar of Black resilience, offer psychological relief.

3. Regular Physical Activity

Exercise helps release endorphins, lowers cortisol, and improves overall mood.

Walking, dancing, and traditional African movement practices promote both physical and emotional well-being.

4. Journaling and Expressive Healing

Writing down thoughts, feelings, and experiences is a therapeutic way to process stress.

Engaging in creative outlets, such as poetry, art, and music, provides emotional release.

5. Accessing Mental Health Care and Therapy

Breaking the stigma around therapy in the Black community is crucial for healing.

Seeking Black therapists or culturally competent mental health providers improves the effectiveness of treatment.

Managing stress is not just about surviving—it is about thriving. African Americans experience higher levels of stress due to systemic oppression, economic challenges, and racialized trauma, but by engaging in mindfulness, building strong support networks, and prioritizing self-care, we can reclaim health and resilience.

ELEMENT 12 – CONNECTION:
BUILDING BELONGING AND SAFE SPACE

Human beings are wired for connection, and social relationships play a critical role in emotional, mental, and physical well-being. For African Americans, the concept of connection has always been a vital survival tool, from the collective strength of enslaved ancestors to the formation of Black-led movements, faith-based institutions, and grassroots organizations that sustain the community, as discussed in the previous chapter. However, systemic oppression, racial discrimination, and historical trauma have disrupted communal bonds, dismantled trust, leaving many Black individuals feeling isolated, disconnected, and emotionally burdened. Strong relationships and social support networks enhance resilience, reduce stress, and promote healing.

By prioritizing connection, African Americans can reclaim a sense of belonging, strengthen social capital, and foster collective well-being, all of which are essential for improving overall health outcomes.

Why Connection is Essential to Whole Health

Enhances mental and emotional well-being, reducing anxiety and depression.

Strengthens the immune system and lowers stress hormones like cortisol.

Increases longevity and reduces the risk of chronic diseases.

Encourages personal growth and professional advancement through mentorship.

Provides a buffer against racial trauma, discrimination, and societal challenges.

Without connection, individuals are more vulnerable to mental health struggles, stress-related illnesses, and a diminished sense of purpose.

Physiological and Psychological Impact of Disconnection

Social Isolation and Mental Health Decline

Research show that social isolation and loneliness are not limited to only increasing the risk of depression and anxiety, but also heart disease, stroke, and even early death.[316]

African Americans are more likely to experience social isolation due to economic barriers, and systemic exclusion.

Disrupted Social Networks and Health Disparities

A strong sense of community can increase health literacy, access to resources, and support for those navigating chronic illnesses.

Black individuals with stronger social ties tend to have improved cardiovascular health and better stress regulation.[317]

The Impact of Racism on Social Belonging

Experiencing racial discrimination leads to social withdrawal, increased cortisol levels, and chronic stress.

Black professionals often face 'code-switching' adjusting behavior to fit into predominantly white spaces leading to additional stress and emotional exhaustion.

The Role of Faith, Spirituality, and Collective Healing

Historically, the Black church has been a central institution providing spiritual, emotional, and tangible resources to the community.

Spiritual practices, including prayer, meditation, and faith-based gatherings, contribute to stress reduction and a stronger sense of belonging.

How Connection and Community Influence Black Health

- **The Power of Collective Healing**—Healing circles, group therapy, and community-based initiatives provide emotional support and validation. Cultural traditions such as storytelling, music, and dance foster intergenerational connections and mental wellness.

- **Economic and Professional Growth**—Networking within Black-owned businesses and organizations increases financial empowerment. Mentorship and collective wealth-building strategies strengthen community resilience.
- **Health Advocacy and Activism**—Black-led health movements, like those championed by organizations such as the Black Panther Party's Free Breakfast Program, have historically provided life-saving resources. Modern public health initiatives focused on African Americans advocate for policy changes that improve access to care and equity.

Undeniably so, the experience of life is enhanced when shared in nurturing and supportive relationships with people we share a connection with. Connection anchors us, holds us accountable, and supports us to the other side of trying times, and celebrates with us when we arrive there. On the flip side, isolation will kill you if you let it. Within an 18-month period of time, I experienced more loss than I thought my soul could possibly bear. I buried both my mother and my maternal grandmother, who primarily raised me. I made the courageous decision to divorce my husband two and a half years after we relocated to the other side of the country during the pandemic. No parents, no husband, no family, and no local friends, just me and God. The grief was unbearable; it was compounded, and it felt unrelenting. I had never felt so alone in my entire life. I cried, and I prayed. I prayed and I cried all in between counseling sessions and grief support groups. As I wrestled with the dark nights of the soul, the spirit within me would not let me give up. I came face-to-face with a fuller understanding that I did not completely comprehend before that time, that God was ALL I needed, until that moment when God was literally ALL I had. I began to surrender and continuously rejoice in the beauty that would one day be on the other side of all that pain, long before it actually arrived. Little by little and bit by bit, God filled my heart with an overflow of joy, and then God kept sending me in-person connections that continue to evolve into community, friendship, and kinship. I found the beauty that arose from my brokenness, and the love of others helped penetrate and dissolve the weight of that unfathomable pain.

Holistic Strategies to Strengthen Connection in the Black Community

1. Rebuild Social Networks

Prioritize deepening relationships with family, friends, and trusted community members.

Engage in intergenerational connections to preserve cultural knowledge and history.

2. Foster Safe Spaces for Emotional Support

Seek Black-centered therapy and support groups to process racial stress and trauma.

Utilize online communities and affinity groups to build meaningful connections.

3. Engage in Collective Healing Practices

Participate in drumming circles, group meditation, and other cultural healing traditions.

Attend cultural festivals, celebrations, and spiritual gatherings to nurture a sense of belonging.

4. Support Black-Owned Businesses and Initiatives

Invest in community-driven businesses that reinvest wealth within Black neighborhoods.

Promote financial literacy and cooperative economics within social circles.

5. Strengthen Political and Health Advocacy

Engage in civic action, grassroots organizing, and health policy reform.

Empower Black youth through mentorship programs and educational initiatives.

Connection is the foundation of health and well-being. When Black individuals cultivate strong relationships, invest in community networks, and engage in cultural traditions, we create a powerful support system that counters systemic oppression and promotes healing. By embracing deep social ties, faith-based resilience, and economic empowerment, the Black community can sustain itself, improve health outcomes, and reclaim wellness for future generations.

Part IV: RECLAIMING BLACK WELLNESS

BONUS ELEMENT – PREVENTION IS POWER:
TAKING CHARGE BEFORE DISEASE TAKES HOLD

Despite the disproportionate rates of chronic disease, morbidity, and mortality among African Americans, disease prevention remains one of the most powerful tools for reclaiming control over health and longevity. The burden of illness is not just physical; it disrupts every aspect of life, draining time, energy, and financial resources, all of which could otherwise be spent on personal fulfillment, family, and economic growth. By prioritizing preventative care, adopting healthy behaviors as a lifestyle, and being proactive in managing health, Black individuals can shift from surviving to thriving. Early detection of disease is great, but protecting your whole health from disease will always be the most ideal.

Each of the 12 Key Wellness Elements previously discussed provides a blueprint for long-term health and resilience. Whether an individual is navigating health imbalances or working to maintain well-being, integrating these principles, from stress management and nutrition to movement and immune strengthening, creates a foundation for lifelong wellness. The key to wellness success lies in the consistency of healthy practices, informed decision-making, and a commitment to valuing self-care as an act of resistance against a system designed to neglect Black health.

Key Preventative Measures: Staying Ahead of Disease

Over the past decade of practicing naturopathic medicine, I have witnessed often enough 3 primary themes within the Black community presenting as self-imposed barriers of seeking out medical attention in a timely fashion. There is the distrust some Black patients have towards doctors in general, justifiably so, considering the long-standing history of abuse on Black bodies. Therefore, avoiding doctor's visits is usually the preferred choice until their bodies loudly (painfully) communicate something different. Then there are those patients who completely distrust the conventional medical model, particularly if the use of herbal and other natural therapies was a long-standing tradition in how their family managed internal ailments, similar to the practices our ancestors relied upon. These individuals are usually self-reliant in navigating the care of their health during perceived problems. In addition to the distrust, there is also an over-reliance on faith for healing, often stimulated by the lack of trust in doctors or conventional medicine. Trusting, believing, and praying to God for a miraculous healing is far easier than going to the doctor. Being driven by such deep-seated mistrust overrides their ability to understand that God has no limitations, that same divine power works through physicians. God has equipped doctors with extensive knowledge, experience, and resources to treat health conditions and help patients make a more informed decision about their health. Ultimately, regardless of the type of distrust/ingrained beliefs, too many Black patients forgo any type of medical care, check-ups, or routine observations. Financial challenges are a very legitimate reason to support their decision to disregard exams, however, that is not always the case for everyone.

Unfortunately, the severe consequences often attached to avoiding regular health exams are not exclusive to distrust, but they can also include any number of reasons, such as: lacking health insurance or managing a demanding schedule of work and/or family obligations, leaving no time for personal healthcare. Regardless of the cause, all can lead to medical emergencies that could otherwise be avoided with routine health checkups and lab evaluations. In such cases, what is seen in many of these patients is more aggressive disease progressions that have been performing damage behind the scenes on a cellular level for months, years, or decades before patients are forced by their ailing bodies to get the disruption or obstruction, resulting in pain, checked out.

Just as I was completing this book, one of my undergraduate classmates from Howard University, Ananda Lewis, a celebrity host of past shows on BET & MTV, was pronounced dead at the age of 52 from Stage 4 Breast Cancer. Diagnosed with Stage 3 cancer in 2019, Ananda reported in interviews that she was utilizing various integrative therapies that were effective while she was being treated. Still, financial limitations and the repercussions of COVID-19 limited her access, prohibiting her from being consistent. Lewis faced the stress of maintaining the livelihood for her and her son, so her focus shifted to survival. With nothing in place to harness the cancer, it eventually spread beyond its localized position and ultimately resulted in her untimely passing. In an interview this year in Essence Magazine, she stated,

"Do everything in your power to avoid my story becoming yours. If I had known what I know now 10 years ago, perhaps I wouldn't have ended up here. I would have been cold plunging, exercising consistently, making sure my vitamin D levels were good, detoxing my body on a monthly and yearly basis, and sleeping better. I would've been doing all the things I've been forced to do now, to keep my body from creating more cancer and remove what it has already made."[318]

Although Ananda was at peace with all her decisions regarding her health, according to her personal values, she still wanted the Black community to learn from her journey. Living from an empowered position means having enough information to make informed decisions about the best ways to manage your health, according to the treatment routes that resonate with you. Do not allow distrust, busy schedules, or self-reliance to manifest into self-neglect. There is nothing enlightening about intentionally choosing not to be aware of the cellular physiology of your own body. Know your lab markers by obtaining a baseline and observing them at least annually if everything appears normal, and more frequently for those values you are working to get in balance or optimize, because the absence of a disease diagnosis is not the same as strong cellular health and vitality. As pointed out in this book, there are so many structural, epigenetic, environmental, and stress factors working against Black wellness that healthy eating and exercise are not enough. Get your labs checked regularly!

Developing a long-term relationship with a trusted primary healthcare provider is one of the most critical steps toward health empowerment. Make this a part of your routine of practicing healthy habits. Regular health screenings serve as a confirmation of wellness progress, a way to identify potential risk factors before they escalate into chronic illnesses, and early detection of disease. The earlier an issue is identified, the greater the chance that your body will respond positively to proven effective interventions (especially if you are incorporating any integrative approaches) and recover more quickly (this can vary from person to person).

Early detection is great; however, your strongest sense of power will always be in disease prevention. Throughout this chapter, I have demonstrated a variety of natural approaches to keep your body in its strongest position or support it back towards better optimization. With disease prevention, you will spend the least amount of money and invest the least amount of time in getting well, and it can all be done in a way that is significantly less disruptive to your life. You may not want to take a few supplements daily, stop eating dessert after dinner every night, or exercise regularly as prevention tactics. Do what is seemingly hard while it is easy. Anything that you can control can always be accomplished with more ease. With a disease diagnosis, you will not have the same flexibility and fluidity of ease when faced with a life-or-death requirement to take multiple medications with potential side effects, see several specialists every month, have debilitating pain, experience a sense of perpetual overwhelm, and have a diminished quality of life. There is nothing easy about managing a body whose ability to function feels more like suffering. I affirm Ananda's closing statement to her interview when she said, "Prevention is the real cure." Let us receive the transparency of sharing her experience and words of wisdom as an opportunity to transform our own health journeys going forward.

Essential Health Screenings for African Americans:

Blood Pressure Monitoring– Measures the pressure in the arteries as the heart pumps. High blood pressure (hypertension) is one of the leading causes of stroke, heart disease, and kidney failure in African Americans. Early detection and management can drastically reduce the risk of cardiovascular complications.

Cholesterol Levels– Unchecked cholesterol contributes to atherosclerosis (plaque buildup in the arteries), heart attacks, and strokes. Routine screening allows for dietary and lifestyle interventions to prevent cardiovascular disease.

Diabetes Screening– Monitoring blood glucose levels regularly can detect prediabetes and prevent its progression to Type 2 diabetes. The Black population makes up 12.1% of diagnosed diabetes cases.[319]

Vitamin D Levels– Due to higher melanin levels, African Americans are at increased risk for vitamin D deficiency, which is linked to risk of weakened immune function, bone loss, and cardiovascular disease.

Serum Iron Levels– Low iron can lead to iron deficiency anemia, which disproportionately affects Black women, causing fatigue, headaches, shortness of breath, rapid or irregular heartbeat, and dizziness.

Ferritin– This measures iron storage and is the most sensitive test to detect iron deficiency.

High-Sensitivity C-Reactive Protein– A key inflammation marker that predicts heart disease risk. African Americans have a higher prevalence of hypertension, stroke, and heart disease, and elevated hs-CRP levels can signal underlying inflammation contributing to these conditions.

Homocysteine– Elevated levels are associated with cardiovascular disease, stroke, and cognitive decline. Since African Americans face a higher risk of hypertension and dementia, monitoring homocysteine levels can help guide nutritional and lifestyle interventions to reduce these risks.

Thyroid Levels– Imbalances (too much or too little) of this hormone can cause a variety of symptoms that impact metabolism, weight, energy, digestion, heart rate, breath rate, temperature sensitivities, mood, and other symptoms, based on a deficiency or excess in its circulation.

Cancer Screenings– Routine screenings such as mammograms, prostate exams, colonoscopies, and cervical screenings are essential for early detection and survival. Black individuals face higher cancer mortality rates, often due to later-stage diagnoses.

Eye Exams– Glaucoma and diabetic retinopathy are leading causes of blindness in African Americans. Regular eye exams help prevent irreversible vision loss.

Dental Check-Ups– Oral health is directly linked to cardiovascular disease, diabetes, and systemic infections. Gum disease disproportionately affects African Americans, making dental care an important aspect of disease prevention.

Complementary/Alternative Providers

Beyond conventional medical screenings, African Americans have the right to seek alternative forms of healthcare consultations and services designed to support their individualized holistic wellness needs. Other practitioners can complement your conventional treatments or, in some cases, work independently of traditional methods. The most important thing to know is that part of your self-care is exercising your options to care that align with your value system.

During slavery in the United States, natural remedies and herbal treatments were not only widely used but were often the preferred method for addressing internal illnesses on plantations. Enslaved Africans brought with them a rich heritage of plant-based healing practices from West Africa, where knowledge of roots, leaves, and barks for medicinal use was deeply embedded in daily life and community care. This ancestral wisdom was adapted and preserved, even under the brutal conditions of enslavement. Enslaved individuals frequently relied on native plants, herbs, and other natural substances to care for one another when formal medical treatment was either unavailable, harmful, or reserved for white plantation owners. These remedies were often more trusted than the interventions offered by white physicians, whose methods were at times harmful and experimental toward Black bodies.

This reliance on natural medicine was born of necessity and was also a powerful act of cultural preservation. Many enslaved people cultivated medicinal gardens in hidden patches or incorporated healing rituals into their spiritual practices. Remedies using plants such as garlic, cayenne, sassafras, and horehound were commonly used to treat digestive issues, infections, and respiratory problems.[320] This healing knowledge was passed down through oral tradition and shaped the foundation of African American folk medicine for generations. Today, reconnecting with these ancestral practices by seeking out naturopathic, herbal, or functional approaches to care is not a new trend; it is a return to a tradition that our ancestors used to survive, resist, and care for each other in the face of oppression.

However, during the time of enslavement, plant medicines were not only culturally familiar to African people but also cheap and easily accessible. Herbal treatments were readily available in gardens, forests, or prepared from household ingredients, offering both physical relief and a form of cultural resistance. Today, accessing natural medicine often requires navigating a commercialized wellness landscape that operates outside of conventional healthcare systems. The very remedies once grown freely now often come at a financial cost, especially when seeking support from formally trained and licensed holistic practitioners, such as naturopathic doctors, chiropractors, acupuncturists, or herbalists.

Still, the value of investing in wellness cannot be overstated. For generations, Black communities have been burdened by disproportionate rates of chronic illness, disability, and premature death, outcomes that steal our vitality, time, and freedom. While building a comprehensive wellness team may require out-of-pocket expenses, particularly in a healthcare system that favors pharmaceutical intervention over prevention, the cost of doing nothing is far greater. Even with insurance, managing illness through the conventional medical model is expensive—financially, emotionally, and physically. Chronic conditions often mean missed workdays, multiple prescriptions, long wait times, and reduced quality of life. Preventative care—rooted in holistic, culturally affirming practices—is not a luxury but a protective strategy. You will always spend less on preventing disease than managing it after it has taken hold of your pockets and, more importantly, your life. Choosing to invest in your health is a powerful act of self-preservation and ancestral alignment. You are definitely worth that investment.

1. Naturopathic Doctors (NDs)

Naturopathic doctors like me are trained in both conventional medical sciences and natural therapies. We use personalized, systems-based approaches to identify imbalances in the body, such as gut health issues, hormonal dysfunction, or metabolic disruptions, and restore optimal function. NDs incorporate clinical nutrition, botanical and herbal medicine, lifestyle counseling, and functional diagnostics to address the root causes of illness.

NDs can provide culturally responsive, preventive care to help manage and reduce the risk of chronic diseases disproportionately affecting Black communities. We are especially valuable for complex, chronic illnesses like gastrointestinal disorders, diabetes, hypertension, and autoimmune conditions. Practitioners often address hidden contributors such as chronic stress, toxic exposures, and food sensitivities to help bring the body back to balance.

Part IV: RECLAIMING BLACK WELLNESS

2. Chiropractors (DCs)

Chiropractors specialize in diagnosing and treating musculoskeletal conditions, particularly through spinal adjustments, posture correction, and rehabilitative exercises.

Many chronic conditions like hypertension, back pain, and headaches are exacerbated by physical stress and tension. Chiropractic care can relieve pain, improve mobility, and support nervous system regulation, which is important in combating the physiological effects of racial stress and health inequities.

3. Acupuncturists (L.Ac. or DACM)

Acupuncturists use thin needles to stimulate specific points on the body to balance energy (Qi), reduce inflammation, and restore function.

Acupuncture sessions can help reduce stress, pain, anxiety, and sleep disorders, issues that are often intensified by systemic inequities. It offers a non-pharmaceutical approach to managing chronic diseases and supporting mental health.

4. Herbalists

Herbalists specialize in the use of plant-based medicines to support healing and balance in the body. They may draw from traditional knowledge of African herbal medicine or Traditional Chinese Medicine, formal education, or apprenticeships.

Herbalists can provide culturally rooted healing approaches using plant-based remedies to support immune health, hormonal balance, inflammation, and stress, key areas contributing to disease disparities among Black populations.

Overcoming Racial Bias in Healthcare: The Necessity of Self-Advocacy

While accessing healthcare is vital, navigating a biased medical system presents significant challenges for Black patients. Studies have repeatedly shown that Black individuals experience medical bias in pain management, diagnostic testing, and treatment recommendations. Black patients are more likely to have their symptoms dismissed, receive delayed diagnoses, or be denied further testing or referrals compared to white patients with identical symptoms. Self-advocacy is a crucial skill to ensure that health concerns are taken seriously and appropriately addressed.

Top 5 Self-Advocacy Strategies:

1. Educate Yourself with Trusted Health Resources

Knowledge is power—understand the latest health screenings, disease prevention, and treatment options guidelines.

Rely on evidence-based sources such as the National Institutes of Health (NIH), Centers for Disease Control and Prevention (CDC), and Black-led health organizations such as the National Medical Association and The Center for Black Health & Equity.

2. Come Prepared to Appointments

Write down all symptoms, concerns, and questions before your visit.

Request clarification on any medical decisions. You have the right to understand your healthcare plan.

3. Demand Thorough Examinations and Second Opinions

If a doctor dismisses your symptoms, insist on further testing or seek a second opinion.

If necessary, bring a trusted friend or family member to appointments.

4. Seek Culturally Competent Providers

Choose Black healthcare professionals or providers trained in culturally competent care whenever possible.

Platforms like BlackDoctor.org and Black Emotional and Mental Health Collective (BEAM) help connect Black patients with trusted providers.

5. Use Your Voice to Respectfully Demand Quality Care

If treatment recommendations feel inadequate, ask direct questions:

"Are there additional tests you can run to rule out any serious conditions?"

"What alternative treatment options are available for my condition?"

"Can you refer me to a specialist or a second opinion?"

If you feel dismissed, document the encounter and escalate concerns to a patient advocate, hospital administration, and/or medical board.

While systemic barriers exist, disease prevention remains one of the most optimal ways to reclaim health and longevity. The 12 Key Wellness Elements help us strategize plans of action designed to enhance health and well-being, specific to the needs of the Black community. By prioritizing healthy lifestyle habits, routine screenings, and self-advocacy in medical settings, Black individuals can stay in control of their wellness and avoid preventable health crises. Health is a birthright, not a privilege, requiring intentional self-investment, proactive care, and a refusal to accept substandard treatment. Whether through traditional medicine, holistic therapies, or community-based health initiatives, the power to thrive lies in taking action today for a healthier tomorrow.

CONCLUSION

While concluding this book, it is important to reaffirm the purpose behind its creation: to examine, with intellectual rigor and cultural clarity, the roots of disease vulnerability within the African American community. Throughout the chapters, we have traced how historical dehumanization, structural racism, and systemic exclusion laid the groundwork for a public health crisis that is too often mischaracterized as individual failure. We have examined how chronic physiological stress, environmental exposures, and intergenerational trauma have shaped the physical and mental health of African Americans. They have done so in ways that are often misunderstood, minimized, or willfully ignored by dominant social narratives and institutions.

This book has sought to disrupt those narratives, particularly the persistent myth of biological inferiority that has been used as a scaffold to justify centuries of exclusion, neglect, and mistreatment. When viewed outside of context, the disproportionate rates of hypertension, diabetes, maternal mortality, and premature death among African Americans might appear to confirm that falsehood. Context tells a different story—one rooted not in deficiency, but in systemic injury, neglect, and conditioned survival.

We have shown that wellness among African Americans cannot be understood solely through the lens of behavior, access, or biology alone. Rather, it must be situated within a broader sociopolitical and historical framework that includes the forced commodification of Black bodies, structural disinvestment, culturally invalidating environments, and an enduring stress load borne from constant negotiation of one's safety, humanity, and dignity while trying to survive. When this comprehensive view is adopted, health disparities no

CONCLUSION

longer read as inevitable—they become intelligible, addressable, and profoundly unjust.

Yet, while the landscape of structural racism is vast, it does not render us powerless. On the contrary, history reveals the extraordinary capacity of African Americans not only to survive but to adapt, create, organize, and resist in ways that foster collective advancement. The field of epigenetics affirms what oral history and cultural memory have long conveyed: that trauma may shape biology, but so too can healing. Our environments matter, and so do the internal conditions we intentionally cultivate within ourselves and our communities.

In this light, wellness must be reclaimed not only as an outcome but as a cultural imperative. It is not merely the absence of disease—it is the presence of agency, context, and self-determination. The everyday choices we make—how we manage stress, nourish our bodies, build community, and assert boundaries—are not small acts. They are, in fact, the building blocks of resistance against systems designed to erode us. And they are within our sphere of influence.

A compelling example from nature illustrates this point. In the 1990s, researchers constructed a sealed ecological system known as Biosphere 2 to observe plant and human life in a controlled environment. Within it, trees grew quickly, but many collapsed before reaching maturity. Scientists discovered the missing variable: wind. In natural environments, wind pressure is essential for trees to develop "stress wood"—dense fibers that help them withstand external forces and grow stronger over time. In the absence of wind, trees become tall but fragile, collapsing under their own weight.

This insight offers a valuable metaphor. The social winds that have shaped the Black experience—forced migration, enslavement, systemic exclusion, and institutional neglect—have certainly tested the strength of our communities. But they have also necessitated the development of a kind of "stress wood": the internal adaptations and cultural fortitudes that make resilience possible. This is not to romanticize our hardship but to underscore the biological and cultural intelligence forged under pressure. Some might refer to this as post-traumatic growth. Our ancestors grew instead of toppling over.

Just like the redwood trees, which grow beyond 300 feet tall by intertwining their roots with those of others, our collective strength lies in our connection. Though their roots are shallow, redwoods do not fall because they hold each other up. This interdependence of redwoods is nature's version of Ubuntu (I am because we are). They can only grow to be the tallest trees on the planet by relying on each other. Likewise, our innermost healing depends not only on individual wellness but also on our capacity to fortify one another through community, shared cultural practices, and collective commitment to thriving.

Still, wellness must begin within. We have already experienced the long, stony road towards equity and systemic barriers being dismantled. Right now, we have the most influence over what we consume, how we manage stress, where we seek support, and how we tend to our bodies and minds. We must prioritize the cultivation of wellness spaces—spaces that affirm our identity, honor our history, and allow us to exhale without fear or performance. This is not a luxury—it is a necessity.

Moving forward, I invite all readers to embrace what is at the heart of this book, a counter-narrative that dismisses inherited myths of inadequacy and instead centers historical context, collective agency, and holistic care. Let us together affirm: we are not broken—we are overburdened. And when those burdens are lifted, even just slightly, we rise. By reclaiming ancestral knowledge, embedding wellness within our cultural frameworks, and advancing both structural reforms and individual practices, African Americans can shift from a paradigm of survival to one of strategic, sustainable thriving.

This book is my invitation: to reframe the conditions of our health, to restore truth where lies once took up permanent residency, and to reimagine what it means to be well—while Black, and beyond.

CONCLUSION

The barriers are real. The trauma is real. The stress is real. But so is our power. Our resilience. Our potential.

Let the wind blow. Let it shape us. And let us stand stronger, rooted, and reaching toward a future together where Black wellness is not an afterthought but a priority to us.

> *"Shadowed beneath Thy hand,*
>
> *May we forever stand,*
>
> *True to our God,*
>
> *True to our Native Land"*
>
> *~ Lift Every Voice and Sing - James Weldon Johnson*

ACKNOWLEDGEMENTS

The writing and research journey on this subject began for me over a decade ago when my then professor encouraged my research topic at a time when the term "racism" was considered taboo to mention out loud, let alone discuss its correlation to cardiovascular disease in African Americans to a medical academic body. I am grateful to Stephanie Draus, ND, for being a gateway and not a barrier to this research. Your support truly made a difference in the trajectory of my scholarship. Years later, my writing Doula, Linda Jones, would meet with me regularly to help me organize my elephant-sized thoughts into more manageable pieces to process and write about. Then came along Raycene Nevils-Karakeçi, my editor, who evolved into a partner in "creative expression." She understood my vision from the start and shared my passion for this project.

I am also grateful for the support of my family, friends, colleagues, and other supportive communities for their presence in my life. Honorable mentions are my life-long mentor, Rev. Cheryl Jones and Baji Daniels, Ph.D., my New Thought spiritual mother. I am thankful for the experience of teaching this critical topic over the past four years to my former medical students as they prepared to become a better generation of physicians. I am also grateful to my patients and clients who have trusted me to guide their journey of wellness, therefore providing me with the opportunity to learn from them as much as they have learned from me. It is indeed a great honor to be repeatedly invited to serve in that capacity. Lastly, but certainly not least, I am grateful to my late grandparents, Leroy and Olevia, whose love and support of me was unwavering throughout their entire lives. Finally, to my late loving mother, Peggy, I can only sum up my words of never-ending love and gratitude for you with, "You were right."

ENDNOTES

Chapter 1

1. Jeffrey Rogers Hummel, "U.S. Slavery and Economic Thought," in *The Concise Encyclopedia of Economics,* ed. David R. Henderson (Liberty Fund, 2008), accessed May 13, 2025, https://www.econlib.org/library/enc/usslaveryandeconomicthought.html. & Jenny B. Wahl, "Slavery in the United States," in The Concise Encyclopedia of Economics, ed. David R. Henderson, Carleton College, accessed May 13, 2025, https://web.mnstate.edu/stutes/econ411/readings/slaves.html & Samuel H. Williamson, "Seven Ways to Compute the Relative Value of a U.S. Dollar Amount, 1790 to Present," Measuring Worth, 2025, accessed May 13, 2025, https://www.measuringworth.com/uscompare/
2. Ibram X. Kendi, *Stamped from the Beginning: The Definitive History of Racist Ideas in America* (New York: Nation Books, 2016), 53.
3. Jacqueline Battalora, *Birth of a White Nation: The Invention of White People and Its Relevance Today* (Houston: Strategic Book Publishing, 2013), 15.
4. Edmund S. Morgan, *American Slavery, American Freedom: The Ordeal of Colonial Virginia* (New York: W. W. Norton & Company, 1975).
5. Ibram X. Kendi, *Stamped from the Beginning: The Definitive History of Racist Ideas in America* (New York: Nation Books, 2016), 53.
6. Jacqueline Battalora, *Birth of a White Nation: The Invention of White People and Its Relevance Today* (Houston: Strategic Book Publishing, 2013), 37.
7. "What caused the Rwandan Genocide? - Susanne Buckley-Zistel," posted June 27, 2023, by TED-Ed, YouTube, 6:21, https://youtu.be/MF7EbUGlaOU?si=Dw1llcdwmnGapoYh & "A History of The Tutsi," posted Nov. 9, 2018, by HomeTeam History, YouTube, 12:57, https://youtu.be/FEXSQmbS54I?si=wibFkrslXDpDHWJ8
8. Harriet A. Washington, *Medical Apartheid: The Dark History of Medical Experimentation on Black Americans from Colonial Times to the Present* (New York: Doubleday, 2006), 32.
9. Charles Caldwell, *Thoughts on the Original Unity of the Human Race* (Louisville: Prentice and Weissinger, 1852), 81, 95-100.
10. Ibid. 76-77
11. Harriet A. Washington, *Medical Apartheid: The Dark History of Medical Experimentation on Black Americans from Colonial Times to the Present* (New York: Doubleday, 2006), 36.

12 Samuel A. Cartwright, *Diseases and Peculiarities of the Negro Race*. (DeBow's Review, 1851), 11, 331-336.
13 Todd L. Savitt, *Medicine and Slavery: The Diseases and Health Care of Blacks in Antebellum Virginia* (Urbana: University of Illinois Press, 2002), 11.
14 Peter Kolchin, *American Slavery, 1619-1877* (New York: Hill and Wang, 2003), 193.
15 Samuel George Morton, *Crania Americana: Or, A Comparative View of the Skulls of Various Aboriginal Nations of North and South America* (Philadelphia: J. Dobson, 1839), 5-6, 264-268.
16 W. Michael Byrd and Linda A. Clayton, *An American Health Dilemma: A Medical History of African Americans and the Problem of Race: Beginnings to 1900*, vol. 1 (New York: Routledge, 2000), 104.
17 Stephen Jay Gould, *The Mismeasure of Man* (New York: W. W. Norton & Company, 1981), 94.
18 Harriet A. Washington, *Medical Apartheid: The Dark History of Medical Experimentation on Black Americans from Colonial Times to the Present* (New York: Doubleday, 2006), 33-34 & Michael Byrd and Linda A. Clayton, An American Health Dilemma: A Medical History of African Americans and the Problem of Race: Beginnings to 1900, vol. 1 (New York: Routledge, 2000), 106-107.
19 Josiah C. Nott and George R. Gliddon, *Types of Mankind: Or, Ethnological Researches Based upon the Ancient Monuments, Paintings, Sculptures, and Crania of Races* (Philadelphia: Lippincott, Grambo & Co., 1854).
20 Geoffrey Galt Harpham, ed., "Theories of Race: An Annotated Anthology of Essays on Race, 1684-1900, part of the "Who's Black and Why?" project, accessed May 13, 2025, https://www.theoriesofrace.com/.
21 Josiah C. Nott and George R. Gliddon, *Types of Mankind: Or, Ethnological Researches Based upon the Ancient Monuments, Paintings, Sculptures, and Crania of Races* (Philadelphia: Lippincott, Grambo & Co., 1854), 135-136.
22 W. Michael Byrd and Linda A. Clayton, *An American Health Dilemma: A Medical History of African Americans and the Problem of Race: Beginnings to 1900*, vol. 1 (New York: Routledge, 2000), 106-107.
23 Kenneth F. Kiple and Virginia H. King, *Another Dimension to the Black Diaspora: Diet, Disease, and Racism* (Cambridge: Cambridge University Press, 1981), 24-31, 71-75.
24 W. Michael Byrd and Linda A. Clayton, *An American Health Dilemma: A Medical History of African Americans and the Problem of Race: Beginnings to 1900*, vol. 1 (New York: Routledge, 2000), 249.
25 Harriet A. Washington, *Medical Apartheid: The Dark History of Medical Experimentation on Black Americans from Colonial Times to the Present* (New York: Doubleday, 2006), 61-65.
26 Hoffman, K. M., Trawalter, S., Axt, J. R., & Oliver, M. N. (2016). "Racial bias in pain assessment and treatment recommendations, and false beliefs about biological differences between blacks and whites." *Proceedings of the National Academy of Sciences*, 113(16), 4296-4301. https://doi.org/10.1073/pnas.1516047113

Endnotes

27 Vyas, D. A., Eisenstein, L. G., & Jones, D. S. (2020). "Hidden in Plain Sight – Reconsidering the Use of Race Correction in Clinical Algorithms." *New England Journal of Medicine*, 383(9), 874-882. https://www.nejm.org/doi/full/10.1056/NEJMms2004740

28 Donna L. Hoyert, Health E-Stat: Maternal Mortality Rates in the United States, 2022, National Center for Health Statistics, Health E-Stats, May 2, 2024, accessed April 25, 2025, https://www.cdc.gov/nchs/data/hestat/maternal-mortality/2022/

Chapter 2

29 World Health Organization, "Retrieved April 1, 2021" Constitution. https://www.who.int/about/who-we-are/constitution

30 Kenneth M. Stampp, *The Peculiar Institution: Slavery in the Ante-Bellum South* (New York: Alfred A. Knopf, 1956), 299.

31 Marcus Rediker, *The Slave Ship: A Human History* (New York: Viking, 2007), 308.

32 Olaudah Equiano, *The Interesting Narrative of the Life of Olaudah Equiano, Or Gustavus Vassa, The African*, 1789, https://www.pbs.org/wgbh/aia/part1/1h320t.html

33 Ibid.

34 Ibid.

35 Encyclopedia Britannica, s.v. "Middle Passage," accessed March 28, 2025, https://www.britannica.com/topic/Middle-Passage-slave-tradeIbid.

36 *Federal Writers' Project: Slave Narrative Project, Vol. 2, Arkansas, Part 6, Quinn-Tuttle.* 1936. Manuscript/Mixed Material. 325 (Laura Thornton) https://www.loc.gov/item/mesn026/.

37 Edward E. Baptist, (2014). *The Half Has Never Been Told: Slavery and the Making of American Capitalism*. Basic Books. p. 140.

38 F. Blaine Rankin-Hill, *A Biohistory of 19th-Century Afro-Americans: The Burial Remains of a Philadelphia Cemetery* (Westport, CT: Bergin & Garvey, 1997), 152.

39 Frederick Douglass, *Narrative of the Life of Frederick Douglass, an American Slave, Written by Himself* (Boston: Anti-Slavery Office, 1845), 55.

40 Harriet A. Jacobs, *Incidents in the Life of a Slave Girl*, ed. Jean Fagan Yellin (Cambridge, MA: Harvard University Press, 1987) 88. Originally published in 1861.

41 Deborah G. White, (1999). *Ar'n't I a woman?: Female slaves in the plantation South*. W. W. Norton & Company. p. 68.

42 Geronimus, A. T. (2013). "Deep integration: Letting the epigenome out of the bottle without losing sight of the structural origins of population health." *American Journal of Public Health*, 103(S1), S56–S63.

43 Sharla M. Fett, *Working Cures: Healing, Health, and Power on Southern Slave Plantations* (Chapel Hill: University of North Carolina Press, 2002), 178.

44 Williams, D. R., & Mohammed, S. A. (2009). "Discrimination and racial disparities in health: Evidence and needed research." *Journal of Behavioral Medicine*, 32(1), 20–47. https://doi.org/10.1007/s10865-008-9185-0

45 Peter Kolchin, *American Slavery*, 1619-1877 (New York: Hill and Wang, 2003), 114.

46 *Federal Writers' Project: Slave Narrative Project, Vol. 4, Georgia, Part 1, Adams-Furr.* 1936. Manuscript/Mixed Material. https://www.loc.gov/item/mesn041/. Pg 3 Rachel Adams Ex-Slave
47 Ibid.
48 Todd L. Savitt, *Medicine and Slavery: The Diseases and Health Care of Blacks in Antebellum Virginia* (Urbana: University of Illinois Press, 2002), 37.
49 W. Michael Byrd and Linda A. Clayton, *An American Health Dilemma: A Medical History of African Americans and the Problem of Race: Beginnings to 1900*, vol. 1 (New York: Routledge, 2000), 225.
50 Harriet A. Jacobs, *Incidents in the Life of a Slave Girl*, ed. Jean Fagan Yellin (Cambridge, MA: Harvard University Press, 1987), 8. Originally published in 1861.
51 Kenneth F. Kiple and Virginia Himmelsteib King, *Another Dimension to the Black Diaspora: Diet, Disease and Racism* (Cambridge: Cambridge University Press, 1981), 80.
52 *Federal Writers' Project: Slave Narrative Project, Vol. 4, Georgia, Part 1, Adams-Furr.* 1936. Manuscript/Mixed Material. https://www.loc.gov/item/mesn041/ Pg 22, 23 Celestia Avery- Ex-Slave.
53 Frederick Douglass, *Narrative of the Life of Frederick Douglass, an American Slave*, Written by Himself (Boston: Anti-Slavery Office, 1845), 96.
54 Todd L. Savitt, *Medicine and Slavery: The Diseases and Health Care of Blacks in Antebellum Virginia* (Urbana: University of Illinois Press, 2002), 90.
55 Massachusetts Institute of Technology: Slavery and Diseases in the Antebellum American South. Retrieved on 12/2/2024. By RA McGuire published 4/8/2020. https://covid-19.mitpress.mit.edu/pub/8flb6457/release/1
56 Kenneth F. Kiple and Virginia Himmelsteib King, *Another Dimension to the Black Diaspora: Diet, Disease and Racism* (Cambridge: Cambridge University Press, 1981), 127-128.
57 Michael L. Blakey and Lesley M. Rankin-Hill, eds., *The Skeletal Biology of the New York African Burial Ground: Volume I, Part I* (Washington, DC: Howard University Press, 2009), 221-267.

Chapter 3

58 Michael A. Gomez, *Exchanging Our Country Marks: The Transformation of African Identities in the Colonial and Antebellum South* (Chapel Hill: University of North Carolina Press, 1998).
59 Sterling Stuckey, *Slave Culture: Nationalist Theory and the Foundations of Black America* (New York: Oxford University Press, 1987), 25.
60 Walter Johnson, *Soul by Soul: Life Inside the Antebellum Slave Market* (Cambridge, MA: Harvard University Press, 1999), 165.
61 Frederick Douglass, Narrative of the Life of Frederick Douglass, an American Slave (Boston: Anti-Slavery Office, 1845), 105.
62 *Federal Writers' Project: Slave Narrative Project, Vol. 14, South Carolina, Part 1, Abrams-Durant.* 1936.. Manuscript/Mixed Material. 5-6, Ezra Adams. https://www.loc.gov/item/mesn141/

Endnotes

63 Albert J. Raboteau, Slave Religion: The "Invisible Institution" in the Antebellum South. New York: Oxford University Press, 2004.
64 Olaudah Equiano, The Interesting Narrative of the Life of Olaudah Equiano, Or Gustavus Vassa, The African, 1789, https://www.pbs.org/wgbh/aia/part1/1h320t.html.
65 Heather Andrea Williams, Help Me to Find My People: The African American Search for Family Lost in Slavery (Chapel Hill: University of North Carolina Press, 2012), 24.
66 Ibid, 12.
67 John Bowlby, A Secure Base: Parent-Child Attachment and Healthy Human Development (New York: Basic Books, 1988).
68 Bessel van der Kolk, The Body Keeps the Score: Brain, Mind, and Body in the Healing of Trauma (New York: Viking, 2014), 182.
69 bell hooks. Belonging: A Culture of Place. New York: Routledge, 2009.
70 Jacqueline Jones, Labor of Love, Labor of Sorrow: Black Women, Work, and the Family from Slavery to the Present (New York: Basic Books, 1985).
71 Captured during a personal visit to Whitney Plantation on 4/6/24024 - formerly enslaved monument narratives - J.F. Boone. Received from the Federal Writers Project.
72 Federal Writers' Project, Slave Narrative Project, Vol. 4, Georgia, Part 1, Adams-Furr, 1936, manuscript/mixed material, 14–15 (Interview with Rev. W. B. Allen), https://www.loc.gov/item/mesn041/.
73 Federal Writers' Project: Slave Narrative Project, Vol. 16, Texas, Part 1, Adams-Duhon. 1936. Manuscript/Mixed Material. 14 (Interview with Andy Anderson) https://www.loc.gov/item/mesn161/.
74 Daina Ramey Berry, The Price for Their Pound of Flesh: The Value of the Enslaved, from Womb to Grave, in the Building of a Nation (Boston: Beacon Press, 2017), 78.
75 "Buck Breaking." Directed by Tariq Nasheed. Chatsworth, CA: King Flex Entertainment, 2021. DVD.
76 Deborah Gray White, Ar'n't I a Woman?: Female Slaves in the Plantation South, rev. ed. (New York: W. W. Norton & Company, 1999), 68.
77 Frantz Fanon, Black Skin, White Masks, trans. Richard Philcox (New York: Grove Press, 2008; originally published 1952).
78 Ralph Ellison, The Collected Essays of Ralph Ellison, ed. John F. Callahan (New York: Modern Library, 1995).
79 Deborah G. White, (1999). Ar'n't I a woman?: Female slaves in the plantation South. W. W. Norton & Company. p. 69.
80 This age varied from plantation to plantation. Children as early as 7 years of age were given various tasks such as tending animals, gardens, taking water to the fields, kitchen and housework. Boys might learn trades like carpentry or blacksmith
81 Captured during a personal visit to Whitney Plantation on 4/6/24024 - formerly enslaved monument narratives - Mary Ann John. Received from the Federal Writers Project.
82 Daina Ramey Berry, The Price for Their Pound of Flesh: The Value of the Enslaved, from Womb to Grave, in the Building of a Nation (Boston: Beacon Press, 2017), 79.

83 Deborah Gray White, *Ar'n't I a Woman?: Female Slaves in the Plantation South*, rev. ed. (New York: W. W. Norton & Company, 1999), 9.

84 *Federal Writers' Project, Slave Narrative Project, Vol. 4, Georgia, Part 1, Adams-Furr*, 1936, manuscript/mixed material, 24-25 (Interview with Celestia Avery), https://www.loc.gov/item/mesn041/.

85 Nell Irvin Painter, The History of White People (New York: W. W. Norton & Company, 2010).

86 Harriet Jacobs, *Incidents in the Life of a Slave Girl*, ed. Jean Fagan Yellin (Cambridge, MA: Harvard University Press, 1987), 77, 28. Originally published 1861.

87 Walter Johnson, *Soul by Soul: Life Inside the Antebellum Slave Market* (Cambridge, MA: Harvard University Press, 1999), 107.

88 Evelyn Nakano Glenn, "Yearning for Lightness: Transnational Circuits in the Marketing and Consumption of Skin Lighteners," *Gender & Society* 22, no. 3 (2008): 281, https://doi.org/10.1177/0891243208316089.

89 David R. Williams and Selina A. Mohammed, "Discrimination and Racial Disparities in Health: Evidence and Needed Research," *Journal of Behavioral Medicine* 32, no. 1 (2009): 20–47, https://doi.org/10.1007/s10865-008-9185-0.

90 Frantz Fanon, *Black Skin, White Masks*, trans. Richard Philcox (New York: Grove Press, 2008; originally published 1952), 11.

91 *Statutes at Large of South Carolina*, vol. 7, ed. Thomas Cooper and David J. McCord (Columbia, SC: A. S. Johnston, 1840), 397.

92 *St. Cloud Democrat.* [volume] (Saint Cloud, Stearns County, Minn.), 26 June 1862. "Chronicling America: Historic American Newspapers". Lib. of Congress. https://chroniclingamerica.loc.gov/lccn/sn83016836/1862-06-26/ed-1/seq-1/

93 *Green-Mountain Freeman.* [volume] (Montpelier, Vt.), 15 Sept. 1853. "Chronicling America: Historic American Newspapers." Lib. of Congress. https://chroniclingamerica.loc.gov/lccn/sn84023209/1853-09-15/ed-1/seq-2/

94 Frederick Douglass, *Narrative of the Life of Frederick Douglass, an American Slave* (Boston: Anti-Slavery Office, 1845), 140,

95 Paulo Freire, *Pedagogy of the Oppressed*, trans. Myra Bergman Ramos (New York: Bloomsbury, 2000; originally published 1970), Chapter 3.

96 Jarvis R. Givens, *Fugitive Pedagogy: Carter G. Woodson and the Art of Black Teaching* (Cambridge, MA: Harvard University Press, 2021), 9.

97 Janet Duitsman Cornelius, *When I Can Read My Title Clear": Literacy, Slavery, and Religion in the Antebellum South* (Columbia: University of South Carolina Press, 1991).

98 Joy James, *Resisting State Violence: Radicalism, Gender, and Race in U.S. Culture* (Minneapolis: University of Minnesota Press, 1996). & Carol Anderson, *The Psychology of Dehumanization: The Legacy of Slavery and Racism in America* (Boston: Beacon Press, 2004).

99 Bessel van der Kolk, *The Body Keeps the Score: Brain, Mind, and Body in the Healing of Trauma* (New York: Viking, 2014), 88.

Endnotes

100 David R. Williams and Selina A. Mohammed, "Discrimination and Racial Disparities in Health: Evidence and Needed Research," *Journal of Behavioral Medicine* 32, no. 1 (2009): 23, https://doi.org/10.1007/s10865-008-9185-0.

PART II

101 Farrell Evans, "How Neighborhoods Used Restrictive Housing Covenants to Block Nonwhite Families," History.com, December 15, 2022, last updated March 2, 2025, accessed December 17, 2024, https://www.history.com/articles/racially-restrictive-housing-covenants.

102 Richard Rothstein, *The Color of Law: A Forgotten History of How Our Government Segregated America* (New York: Liveright Publishing Corporation, 2017) 63-67.

103 Ibid.

104 Cesar O. Estien, Christine E. Wilkinson, Rachel Morello-Frosch, and Christopher J. Schell, "Historical Redlining Is Associated with Disparities in Environmental Quality across California," *Environmental Science & Technology Letters* 11, no. 2 (2024): 54-59, https://doi.org/10.1021/acs.estlett.3c00870.

105 National Center for Chronic Disease Prevention and Health Promotion (US) Office on Smoking and Health, Community Health and Economic Prosperity: Engaging Businesses as Stewards and Stakeholders—A Report of the Surgeon General (Washington, DC: U.S. Department of Health and Human Services, 2021), chap. 2, https://www.ncbi.nlm.nih.gov/books/NBK568862/.

106 Robert R. Callis, "Younger Householders Drove Rebound in U.S. Homeownership," U.S. Census Bureau, July 25, 2023, https://www.census.gov/library/stories/2023/07/younger-householders-drove-rebound-in-homeownership.html.

107 Junia Howell and Elizabeth Korver-Glenn, Appraised: The Persistent Evaluation of White Neighborhoods as More Valuable Than Communities of Color (Washington University in St. Louis, November 2022), https://nationalfairhousing.org/wp-content/uploads/2022/11/2022-11-2_Howell-and-Korver-Glenn-Appraised.pdf.

108 Julia Craven, "Eviction Is One of the Biggest Health Risks Facing Black Children," New America, December 7, 2023, https://www.newamerica.org/better-life-lab/articles/eviction-health-risks-black-children/

109 David R. Williams, "Why Discrimination Is a Health Issue," Robert Wood Johnson Foundation, October 24, 2017, https://www.rwjf.org/en/insights/blog/2017/10/discrimination-is-a-health-issue.html.

110 Jason Richardson, Bruce Mitchell, and Juan Franco, Shifting Neighborhoods: Gentrification and Cultural Displacement in American Cities (Washington, DC: National Community Reinvestment Coalition, 2019), https://ncrc.org/gentrification/.

111 Arline T. Geronimus, *Weathering: The Extraordinary Stress of Ordinary Life in an Unjust Society* (New York: Little, Brown Spark, 2023), 194-220.

112 Ibid.

113 Brittany Davis et al., "Conceptualizing Gentrification-Induced Social and Cultural Displacement and Place Identity Among Longstanding Black Residents," *Journal of Black Studies* 54, no. 1 (2023): 3-24, https://doi.org/10.1177/00219347231166097

114 U.S. Census Bureau, "Nearly Half of Renter Households Are Cost-Burdened, Proportions Differ by Race," Press Release Number CB24-150, September 12, 2024, https://www.census.gov/newsroom/press-releases/2024/renter-households-cost-burdened-race.html.
115 James Krieger and Donna L. Higgins, "Housing and Health: Time Again for Public Health Action," *American Journal of Public Health* 92, no. 5 (May 2002): 758–768, https://doi.org/10.2105/AJPH.92.5.758.
116 https://douglassclt.org/aboutus/#origins. Accessed on 3/25/25.
117 EdBuild, $23 Billion (February 2019), https://edbuild.org/content/23-billion/full-report.pdf
118 National Center for Education Statistics, NAEP Reading: National Achievement-Level Results, U.S. Department of Education, 2022, https://www.nationsreportcard.gov/reading/nation/achievement/
119 Donald J. Hernandez, Double Jeopardy: How Third-Grade Reading Skills and Poverty Influence High School Graduation (Baltimore: Annie E. Casey Foundation, 2011), https://www.aecf.org/resources/double-jeopardy.
120 Begin to Read Literacy Statistics https://www.begintoread.com/research/literacystatistics.html & Caroline Wolf Harlow, Education and Correctional Populations, Bureau of Justice Statistics Special Report (Washington, DC: U.S. Department of Justice, Office of Justice Programs, January 2003), https://bjs.ojp.gov/content/pub/pdf/ecp.pdf
121 Mark R. Warren, *Willful Defiance: The Movement to Dismantle the School-to-Prison Pipeline* (New York: Oxford University Press, 2021).
122 Paul Hemez, John J. Brent, and Thomas J. Mowen, "Exploring the School-to-Prison Pipeline: How School Suspensions Influence Incarceration During Young Adulthood," *Youth Violence and Juvenile Justice* 18, no. 3 (July 2020): 235–255, https://doi.org/10.1177/1541204019880945.
123 Institute of Education Sciences, "Grow-your-own to Diversify the Teacher Workforce: Examining Recruitment Policies and Pathways to Recruit More Black Teachers," IES Blog, February 16, 2022, https://ies.ed.gov/learn/blog/grow-your-own-diversify-teacher-workforce-examining-recruitment-policies-and-pathways-recruit-more.
124 Nattanicha Chairassamee, Kanokwan Chancharoenchai, and Wuthiya Saraithong, "Getting There: How Commuting Time and Distance Impact Students' Health," *PLOS ONE* 19, no. 12 (2024): e0314687, https://doi.org/10.1371/journal.pone.0314687.
125 Joshua Aronson and Matthew S. McGlone, "Stereotype and Social Identity Threat," in *The Handbook of Prejudice, Stereotyping, and Discrimination*, ed. Todd D. Nelson (New York: Psychology Press, 2009), 153–178.
126 CBS San Francisco, "Oakland Schools Report Fewer Dropouts, Higher Reading Levels With ‹Restorative Justice›," CBS News, January 14, 2015, https://www.cbsnews.com/sanfrancisco/news/oakland-schools-report-fewer-dropouts-higher-reading-levels-with-new-approach-to-discipline-oakland-unified-school-district-edna-brewer-middle-school/.

Endnotes

127 Renee E. Walker, Christopher R. Keane, and Jessica G. Burke, "Disparities and Access to Healthy Food in the United States: A Review of Food Deserts Literature," *Health & Place* 16, no. 5 (2010): 876-884, https://doi.org/10.1016/j.healthplace.2010.04.013.

128 Harvesters Community Food Network, "Why Hunger Impacts Black Communities at a Higher Rate," Harvesters, January 2025, https://www.harvesters.org/why-hunger-impacts-black-communities-at-a-higher-rate.

129 Jason P. Block, Richard A. Scribner, and Karen B. DeSalvo, "Fast Food, Race/Ethnicity, and Income: A Geographic Analysis," *American Journal of Preventive Medicine* 27, no. 3 (October 2004): 211-217, https://doi.org/10.1016/j.amepre.2004.06.007

130 U.S. Department of Health & Human Services, Office of Minority Health, "Diabetes and Black/African Americans," accessed January 30, 2025, https://minorityhealth.hhs.gov/diabetes-and-blackafrican-americans.

131 KFF. "How History Has Shaped Racial and Ethnic Health Disparities: A Timeline of Policies and Events." Last modified July 2021. https://www.kff.org/how-history-has-shaped-racial-and-ethnic-health-disparities-a-timeline-of-policies-and-events/

132 U.S. Department of Health and Human Services, Office of the Assistant Secretary for Planning and Evaluation (ASPE), Health Insurance Coverage and Access to Care Among Black Americans, June 2024, https://aspe.hhs.gov/sites/default/files/documents/4fc0ddbcee8d583d57e399dad6201536/aspe-coverage-access-black-americans-ib.pdf.

133 Jamila Michener and Jerel Ezell, "Structural Racism in Historical and Modern US Health Care Policy," *Health Affairs* 41, no. 2 (February 2022): 187-194, https://doi.org/10.1377/hlthaff.2021.01466.

134 American Cancer Society, "New ACS Study Shows Cancer Mortality Rates Among Black People Declining, but Remain Higher Than Other Racial and Ethnic Groups," news release, February 20, 2025, accessed March 3, 2025, https://www.cancer.org/

135 Centers for Disease Control and Prevention. Pregnancy-Related Deaths: Data From Maternal Mortality Review Committees in 38 U.S. States, 2020. Last modified May 15, 2024. https://www.cdc.gov/maternal-mortality/php/data-research/index.html.

136 Megan E. Morris et al., "Perspectives of Black Patients on Racism Within Emergency Care," *JAMA Health Forum* 5, no. 3 (2024): e240046, https://jamanetwork.com/journals/jama-health-forum/fullarticle/2816056.

137 Kelly M. Hoffman, Sophie Trawalter, John R. Axt, and M. Norman Oliver, "Racial Bias in Pain Assessment and Treatment Recommendations, and False Beliefs About Biological Differences Between Blacks and Whites," *Proceedings of the National Academy of Sciences of the United States of America* 113, no. 16 (2016): 4296-4301, https://doi.org/10.1073/pnas.1516047113.

138 Knox H. Todd, Thomas P. Deaton, Angela P. D'Adamo, and Lawrence Goe, "Ethnicity and Analgesic Practice," *Annals of Emergency Medicine* 35, no. 1 (2000): 11-16.

139 Thomas D. Sequist et al., "Differences in Specialist Consultations for Cardiovascular Disease by Race, Ethnicity, Gender, Insurance Status, and Site of Primary Care," *Circulation* 119, no. 18 (2009): 2463–2470, https://doi.org/10.1161/CIRCULATIONAHA.108.825133

140 Gladys Velarde et al., "Locking the Revolving Door: Racial Disparities in Cardiovascular Disease," *Journal of the American Heart Association* 12, no. 8 (2023): e025271, https://doi.org/10.1161/JAHA.122.025271.

141 Hall, William J., et al. "Implicit Racial/Ethnic Bias Among Health Care Professionals and Its Influence on Health Care Outcomes: A Systematic Review." *American Journal of Public Health* 105, no. 12 (2015): e60–e76. https://doi.org/10.2105/AJPH.2015.302903

142 Dakin Andone, "A Black Doctor Died of Covid-19 Weeks after Accusing Hospital Staff of Racist Treatment," CNN, updated December 25, 2020, accessed January 28, 2025, https://www.cnn.com/2020/12/24/us/black-doctor-susan-moore-covid-19/index.html.

143 Tobi Thomas, "NHS Pilot Uses Virtual Reality to Tackle Racism and Discrimination among Staff," The Guardian, September 22, 2024, accessed March 28, 2025, https://www.theguardian.com/society/2024/sep/22/nhs-pilot-uses-virtual-reality-to-tackle-racism-and-discrimination-among-staff. & TIDES Study, Tackling Inequalities and Discrimination Experiences in Health Services, accessed March 28, 2025, https://tidesstudy.com/.

144 Marianne Bertrand and Sendhil Mullainathan, "Are Emily and Greg More Employable than Lakisha and Jamal? A Field Experiment on Labor Market Discrimination," *American Economic Review* 94, no. 4 (2004): 991–1013, https://doi.org/10.1257/0002828042002561.

145 Dove, The CROWN Act: Research Studies, accessed February 26, 2024, https://www.thecrownact.com/research-studies

146 National Institutes of Health, "Hair Straightener Use and Risk of Uterine Cancer," *NIH Research Matters*, October 17, 2022, accessed February 26, 2024, https://www.nih.gov/news-events/news-releases/hair-straightening-chemicals-associated-higher-uterine-cancer-risk

147 Valerie Wilson and Melat Kassa, "Black Workers Face Two of the Most Lethal Preexisting Conditions for Coronavirus—Racism and Economic Inequality," *Economic Policy Institute*, June 1, 2020, accessed April 25, 2025, https://www.epi.org/publication/black-workers-covid/

148 Marmot, Michael G., Henry Bosma, Harry Hemingway, Eric Brunner, and Stephen Stansfeld. "Contribution of Job Control and Other Risk Factors to Social Variations in Coronary Heart Disease Incidence." *The Lancet* 337, no. 8754 (1991): 1387–1393. https://doi.org/10.1016/0140-6736(91)93068-K.

149 Coqual (formerly Center for Talent Innovation), Being Black in Corporate America: An Intersectional Exploration (September 2020), https://coqual.org/wp-content/uploads/2020/09/CoqualBeingBlackinCorporateAmerica090720-1.pdf

Endnotes

150 Ibid.
151 National Education Association, "Educational Attainment, Income and Earnings, and Unemployment," accessed March 24, 2025, https://www.nea.org/resource-library/educational-attainment-income-and-earnings-and-unemployment
152 Ibid.
153 National Black Worker Center. "Policy." Accessed March 28, 2025. https://nationalblackworkercenters.org/policy/
154 California Task Force to Study and Develop Reparation Proposals for African Americans, Chapter 10: Stolen Labor and Hindered Opportunity, in Final Report, June 29, 2023, 207, https://oag.ca.gov/system/files/media/ch10-ca-reparations.pdf
155 Board of Governors of the Federal Reserve System, Disparities in Wealth by Race and Ethnicity in the 2019 Survey of Consumer Finances, September 28, 2020, accessed February 10, 2025, https://www.federalreserve.gov/econres/notes/feds-notes/disparities-in-wealth-by-race-and-ethnicity-in-the-2019-survey-of-consumer-finances-20200928.htm
156 Andre M. Perry, Jonathan Rothwell, and David Harshbarger, The Devaluation of Assets in Black Neighborhoods: The Case of Residential Property, Brookings Institution, November 27, 2018, accessed January 31, 2025, https://www.brookings.edu/articles/devaluation-of-assets-in-black-neighborhoods/
157 City of Evanston. "Evanston Local Reparations." Accessed March 28, 2025. https://www.cityofevanston.org/government/city-council/reparations & Rachel Treisman, "In Likely First, Chicago Suburb of Evanston Approves Reparations for Black Residents," NPR, March 23, 2021, accessed March 28, 2025, https://www.npr.org/2021/03/23/980277688/in-likely-first-chicago-suburb-of-evanston-approves-reparations-for-black-reside
158 Daniel S. Grossman and David J.G. Slusky, "The Effect of an Increase in Lead in the Water System on Fertility and Birth Outcomes: The Case of Flint, Michigan," Working Paper Series in Theoretical and Applied Economics 201703, University of Kansas, Department of Economics, August 7, 2017, https://researchrepository.wvu.edu/cgi/viewcontent.cgi?article=1017&context=econ_working-pape
159 Steve Wing and Jill Johnston, Industrial Hog Operations in North Carolina Disproportionately Impact African-Americans, Hispanics and American Indians, Department of Epidemiology, University of North Carolina at Chapel Hill, August 29, 2014, accessed April 25, 2025, https://ncnewsline.com/wp-content/uploads/2014/09/UNC-Report.pdf
160 Sarah Unninayar, "Racial, Ethnic Minorities and Low-Income Groups in U.S. Exposed to Higher Levels of Air Pollution," Harvard T.H. Chan School of Public Health, January 12, 2022, accessed January 31, 2025, https://www.hsph.harvard.edu/news/racial-ethnic-minorities-low-income-groups-u-s-air-pollution/
161 American Lung Association. "Disparities in the Impact of Air Pollution." Accessed February 21, 2025. https://www.lung.org/clean-air/outdoors/who-is-at-risk/disparities

162 James Pasley, "Inside Louisiana's Horrifying 'Cancer Alley,' an 85-Mile Stretch of Pollution and Environmental Racism That's Now Dealing with Some of the Highest Coronavirus Death Rates in the Country," Business Insider, April 10, 2020, accessed February 21, 2025, https://www.businessinsider.com/louisiana-cancer-alley-photos-oil-refineries-chemicals-pollution-2019-11

163 Kat Stafford (The Associated Press), "Black Children Are More Likely to Have Asthma. Where They Live Makes a Difference," *Las Vegas Sun*, May 25, 2023, 7.

164 Vivek Shandas, Jeremy Hoffman, Nicholas Pendleton, and David M. Mills, "The Effects of Historical Housing Policies on Resident Exposure to Intra-Urban Heat: A Study of 108 U.S. Urban Areas," *Climate*, vol. 8, no. 1 (2020): 12, https://doi.org/10.3390/cli8010012.

165 Allan Ndovu et al., "Spatial Variation in the Association between Extreme Heat Events and Warm Season Pediatric Acute Care Utilization: A Small-Area Assessment of Multiple Health Conditions and Environmental Justice Implications in California (2005–2019)," *Environmental Health Perspectives* 133, no. 1 (January 2025): 017010, https://doi.org/10.1289/EHP14236

166 Jill Rosenthal, Allie Schneider, Hailey Gibbs, and Mariam Rashid, "How Federal Investments in Safe Drinking Water Infrastructure Are Improving Public Health," *Center for American Progress*, February 5, 2024, accessed March 29, 2025, https://www.americanprogress.org/article/how-federal-investments-in-safe-drinking-water-infrastructure-are-improving-public-health/

167 New York Civil Liberties Union. "A Closer Look at Stop-and-Frisk in NYC." December 12, 2022. Accessed March 28, 2025. https://www.nyclu.org/data/closer-look-stop-and-frisk-nyc

168 Jacob Bor et al., "Police Killings and Their Spillover Effects on the Mental Health of Black Americans: A Population-Based, Quasi-Experimental Study," *The Lancet* 392, no. 10144 (July 28, 2018): 302–310, https://doi.org/10.1016/S0140-6736(18)31130-9.

169 Philip M. Stinson and Chloe A. Wentzlof, "On-Duty Shootings: Police Officers Charged with Murder or Manslaughter, 2005–2019," *Police Integrity Research Group*, Bowling Green State University, 2019, accessed January 28, 2025, https://www.bgsu.edu/content/dam/BGSU/health-and-human-services/document/Criminal-Justice-Program/policeintegritylostresearch/-9-On-Duty-Shootings-Police-Officers-Charged-with-Murder-or-Manslaughter.pdf

170 Richard A. Oppel Jr., "Fatal Police Shootings of Unarmed Black People Reveal Troubling Patterns," NPR, January 25, 2021, accessed January 28, 2025, https://www.npr.org/2021/01/25/956177021/fatal-police-shootings-of-unarmed-black-people-reveal-troubling-patterns

171 Amber Elliott, "Exclusive: New Renderings Show MacGregor Park's $57.5 Million Transformation. Houston Chronicle, March 26 2025, accessed March 31, 2025, https://www.houstonchronicle.com/lifestyle/article/macgregor-park-renderings-20241718.php

172 Robert D. Bullard, "A Call for Transportation Justice Now!" Dr. Robert Bullard, accessed April 27, 2025, https://drrobertbullard.com/a-call-for-transportation-justice-now/

Endnotes

173 Congressional Black Caucus Foundation, New Routes to Equity: The Future of Transportation in the Black Community (Washington, D.C.: Congressional Black Caucus Foundation, October 2020), https://www.cbcfinc.org/wp-content/uploads/2020/10/NewRoutestoEquity-Final5.pdf

174 Krisda H. Chaiyachati et al., "Association of Rideshare-Based Transportation Services and Missed Primary Care Appointments: A Clinical Trial," JAMA Internal Medicine 178, no. 3 (2018): 383-389, https://doi.org/10.1001/jamainternmed.2017.8336.

175 Chicago Transit Authority, "CTA President Carter, FTA Deputy Administrator Vanterpool, Mayor Johnson, and Other Officials Announce Finalization of $1.9 Billion Funding for Transformational Red Line Extension Project," last modified January 10, 2025, accessed March 3, 2025 https://www.transitchicago.com/cta-president-carter-fta-deputy-administrator-vanterpool-mayor-johnson-and-other-officials-announce-finalization-of-19-billion-funding-for-transformational-red-line-extension-project-/

176 Equal Justice Initiative, "Report Documents Racial Bias in Coverage of Crime by Media," last modified December 16, 2021, https://eji.org/news/report-documents-racial-bias-in-coverage-of-crime-by-media/

177 Jamelle Bouie, "The Dangerous Racialization of Crime in U.S. News Media," Center for American Progress, August 29, 2018, accessed March 31, 2025, https://www.americanprogress.org/article/dangerous-racialization-crime-u-s-news-media/

178 Joy DeGruy, Post Traumatic Slave Syndrome: America's Legacy of Enduring Injury and Healing (Milwaukie, OR: Uptone Press, 2005). Pg. 77.

179 Effua E. Sosoo, Destiny L. Bernard, and Enrique W. Neblett, "The Influence of Internalized Racism on the Relationship Between Discrimination and Anxiety," Cultural Diversity and Ethnic Minority Psychology 26, no. 4 (2020): 570-580, https://doi.org/10.1037/cdp0000320.

180 Mouzon, Dawne M., and Jamila S. McLean. 2016. "Internalized Racism and Mental Health among African-Americans, US-Born Caribbean Blacks, and Foreign-Born Caribbean Blacks." Ethnicity & Health 22 (1): 36-48. doi:10.1080/13557858.2016.1196652.

181 Danice L. Brown and Daniel J. Segrist, "African American Career Aspirations: Examining the Relative Influence of Internalized Racism," Journal of Career Development 43, no. 2 (2016): 177-189, https://doi.org/10.1177/0894845315586256

182 Sherri Gardner, "New Black Studies Curriculum Expands Access to Culturally-Responsive Learning," Teachers College, Columbia University, August 7, 2024, accessed March 31, 2025, https://www.tc.columbia.edu/articles/2024/august/new-black-studies-curriculum-expands-access-to-culturally-responsive-learning/

Chapter 4

183 George M. Slavich and Michael R. Irwin, "From Stress to Inflammation and Major Depressive Disorder: A Social Signal Transduction Theory of Depression," Psychological Bulletin 140, no. 3 (2014): 780, https://doi.org/10.1037/a0035302

184 Arline T. Geronimus et al., "Early Life Adversity and Inflammation in African Americans and Whites in the Midlife in the United States Survey," *Psychosomatic Medicine* 72, no. 7 (2010): 694, https://doi.org/10.1097/PSY.0b013e3181e341e1
185 David R. Williams and Selina A. Mohammed, "Racism and Health I: Pathways and Scientific Evidence," *American Behavioral Scientist* 57, no. 8 (2013): 1153, https://doi.org/10.1177/0002764213487340
186 George M. Slavich and Michael R. Irwin, "From Stress to Inflammation and Major Depressive Disorder: A Social Signal Transduction Theory of Depression," *Psychological Bulletin* 140, no. 3 (2014): 778, https://doi.org/10.1037/a0035302
187 Arline T. Geronimus, *Weathering: The Extraordinary Stress of Ordinary Life in an Unjust Society* (New York: Little, Brown Spark, 2023), 27.
188 Stacy S. Drury et al., "The Association of Telomere Length With Family Violence and Disruption," *Pediatrics* 134, no. 1 (2014): e128, https://doi.org/10.1542/peds.2013-3415. & Arline T. Geronimus et al., "Do US Black Women Experience Stress-Related Accelerated Biological Aging?," *Human Nature* 21, no. 1 (2010): 19, https://doi.org/10.1007/s12110-010-9078-0
189 Cheryl L. Woods-Giscombé, "Superwoman Schema: African American Women's Views on Stress, Strength, and Health," *Qualitative Health Research* 20, no. 5 (2010): 668–683, https://doi.org/10.1177/1049732310361892
190 David R. Williams and Selina A. Mohammed, "Racism and Health I: Pathways and Scientific Evidence," American Behavioral Scientist 57, no. 8 (2013): 1153, https://doi.org/10.1177/0002764213487340
191 Kirsten Bibbins-Domingo et al., "Racial Differences in Incident Heart Failure Among Young Adults," New England Journal of Medicine 360, no. 12 (2009): 1179–1190, https://www.nejm.org/doi/full/10.1056/NEJMoa0807265
192 National Institutes of Health, "Racial Disparities in Stroke Incidence and Death," NIH Research Matters, June 21, 2016, Accessed May 6, 2025, https://www.nih.gov/news-events/nih-research-matters/racial-disparities-stroke-incidence-death
193 Antoinette T. Forde et al., "Discrimination and Hypertension Risk Among African Americans in the Jackson Heart Study," Hypertension, no. 3 (2020): 715-723.
194 Sherman A. James, "John Henryism and the Health of African-Americans," *Culture, Medicine and Psychiatry* 18, no. 2 (June 1994): 163–182, https://doi.org/10.1007/BF01379448.
195 Arline T. Geronimus, *Weathering: The Extraordinary Stress of Ordinary Life in an Unjust Society* (New York: Little, Brown Spark, 2023), 190.
196 Christian B. *Oral History*, April 11, 2018, "Underrepresented Voices Oral History Collection," Stuart A. Rose Manuscript, Archives, and Rare Book Library, Emory University.
197 Ibid.
198 Metabolic Syndrome is characterized by meeting at least 4 of the following criteria: Waist circumference >35 for females and >40 for males Abdominal obesity, Triglycerides > 150; HDL cholesterol <50 for women and < 40 for men; Blood Pressure >/= 135/85 or on anti-hypertensive medication; Glucose > 100.

Endnotes

199 Cheryl D. Fryar, Margaret D. Carroll, and Joseph Afful, "Prevalence of Overweight, Obesity, and Severe Obesity Among Adults Aged 20 and Over: United States, 1960-1962 Through 2017-2018," *NCHS Health E-Stats*, December 2020, https://www.cdc.gov/nchs/data/hestat/obesity-adult-17-18/obesity-adult.htm
200 https://diabetes.org/about-diabetes/statistics/about-diabetes
The rates of diagnosed diabetes in adults by race/ethnic background are:
12.1% of non-Hispanic Black adults
6.9% of non-Hispanic White adults
201 U.S. Department of Health and Human Services Office of Minority Health https://minorityhealth.hhs.gov/diabetes-and-blackafrican-americans
202 Ibid.
203 Arline T. Geronimus, *Weathering: The Extraordinary Stress of Ordinary Life in an Unjust Society* (New York: Little, Brown Spark, 2023), 46-49.
204 A. Alotiby, "Immunology of Stress: A Review Article," *Journal of Clinical Medicine* 13, no. 21 (October 25, 2024): 6394, https://doi.org/10.3390/jcm13216394
205 Snežana Vignjević Petrinović, Milena S. Milošević, Dragana Marković, and Siniša Momčilović, "Interplay Between Stress and Cancer—A Focus on Inflammation," *Frontiers in Physiology* 14 (2023): 1119095, https://doi.org/10.3389/fphys.2023.1119095
206 American Cancer Society, "New ACS Study Shows Cancer Mortality Rates Among Black People Declining, but Remain Higher Than Other Racial and Ethnic Groups," news release, February 20, 2025, accessed March 3, 2025, https://www.cancer.org/
207 Duke University Health System, "Social Stress Factors Drive Cancer Mechanisms That Help Explain Racial Disparities," last updated June 13, 2022, accessed March 3, 2025, https://corporate.dukehealth.org/news/social-stress-factors-drive-cancer-mechanisms-help-explain-racial-disparities
208 Sumin Dai et al., "Chronic Stress Promotes Cancer Development," *Frontiers in Oncology* 10 (2020): 1492, https://doi.org/10.3389/fonc.2020.01492.
209 Arline T. Geronimus, *Weathering: The Extraordinary Stress of Ordinary Life in an Unjust Society* (New York: Little, Brown Spark, 2023), 64-79.
210 Ibid 75-76.
211 Neha Singh et al., "Inflammation and Cancer," *Annals of African Medicine* 18, no. 3 (2019): 121-126, https://doi.org/10.4103/aam.aam_56_18
212 The ASCO Post Staff, "Black Patients With Triple-Negative Breast Cancer May Be Less Likely to Receive Immunotherapy Compared With White Patients," The ASCO Post, September 24, 2024, accessed February 27, 2025, https://ascopost.com/news/september-2024/black-patients-with-triple-negative-breast-cancer-may-be-less-likely-to-receive-immunotherapy-compared-with-white-patients/
213 Lisa Armstrong, "Black Women Are More Likely to Experience Infertility Than White Women. They're Less Likely to Get Help, Too," *The Guardian*, December 10, 2023, accessed November 30, 2024, https://www.theguardian.com/us-news/2023/dec/10/black-women-infertility-causes-treatment-inequity-healthcare

214 Pablo A. Nepomnaschy et al., "Cortisol Levels and Very Early Pregnancy Loss in Humans," *Proceedings of the National Academy of Sciences of the United States of America* 103, no. 10 (2006): 3938-3942, https://doi.org/10.1073/pnas.0511183103

215 Centers for Disease Control and Prevention, "Working Together to Reduce Black Maternal Mortality," last reviewed April 3, 2024, accessed April 18, 2025, https://www.cdc.gov/womens-health/features/maternal-mortality.html. https://www.cdc.gov/nchs/data/hestat/maternal-mortality/2022/maternal-mortality-rates-2022

216 Rochester Regional Health, "African American Women and Preeclampsia: What the Data Tells Us," April 11, 2023, accessed January 4, 2025, https://www.rochesterregional.org/hub/preeclampsia-risk-african-american-women & Laura Williamson, "Preeclampsia May Double a Woman's Chances for Later Heart Failure," *American Heart Association News*, August 24, 2020, accessed January 4, 2025, https://www.heart.org/en/news/2020/08/24/preeclampsia-may-double-a-womans-chances-for-later-heart-failure

217 Angela Johnson, "Sisters in Loss," The Root, May 6, 2022, accessed May 30, 2025, https://www.theroot.com/organizations-that-support-black-mothers-and-caregivers-1848891981/slides/2.

218 Joanna Almeida et al., "Racial/Ethnic Inequities in Low Birth Weight and Preterm Birth: The Role of Multiple Forms of Stress," *Maternal and Child Health* Journal 22, no. 8 (August 2018): 1154-1163, https://doi.org/10.1007/s10995-018-2500-7

219 Centers for Disease Control and Prevention, Health, United States, 2008: *With Special Feature on the Health of Young Adults*, accessed March 3, 2021, https://www.cdc.gov/nchs/data/hus/hus08.pdf

220 Arline T. Geronimus, Weathering: The Extraordinary Stress of Ordinary Life in an Unjust Society (New York: Little, Brown Spark, 2023), 101-102. Weathering is exposure to cumulative social and economic disadvantages across the life course lead to acceleration of normal aging processes and earlier onset of diseases for Black Americans compared with White Americans.

221 Bruce S. McEwen, Carla Nasca, and Jason D. Gray, "Stress Effects on Neuronal Structure: Hippocampus, Amygdala, and Prefrontal Cortex," *Neuropsychopharmacology* 41, no. 1 (2016): 3-23, https://doi.org/10.1038/npp.2015.171

222 Eleni Palpatzis et al., "Lifetime Stressful Events Associated with Alzheimer's Pathologies, Neuroinflammation and Brain Structure in a Risk Enriched Cohort," *Annals of Neurology*, first published March 11, 2024, https://doi.org/10.1002/ana.26881

223 National Institute on Aging, "Data Shows Racial Disparities in Alzheimer's Disease Diagnosis Between Black and White Research Study Participants," December 16, 2021, accessed January 3, 2025, https://www.nia.nih.gov/news/data-shows-racial-disparities-alzheimers-disease-diagnosis-between-black-and-white-research

224 Renée Chen et al., "Racial Disparities in Cognitive Function Among Middle-Aged and Older Adults: The Roles of Cumulative Stress Exposures Across the Life Course," *The Journals of Gerontology: Series A, Biological Sciences and Medical Sciences* 77, no. 2 (2022): 357-364, https://doi.org/10.1093/gerona/glab099

Endnotes

225 David R. Williams and Selina A. Mohammed, "Discrimination and Racial Disparities in Health: Evidence and Needed Research," *Journal of Behavioral Medicine* 32, no. 1 (2009): 20-47, https://doi.org/10.1007/s10865-008-9185-0
226 Brett J. Peters, Nickola C. Overall, and Jeremy P. Jamieson, "Physiological and Cognitive Consequences of Suppressing and Expressing Emotion in Dyadic Interactions," International Journal of Psychophysiology 94, no. 1 (October 2014): 100-107, https://www.psych.rochester.edu/research/jamiesonlab/wp-content/uploads/2014/01/peters.pdf
227 Mary-Frances Winters, *Black Fatigue: How Racism Erodes the Mind, Body, and Spirit* (Oakland, CA: Berrett-Koehler Publishers, 2020).
228 Joy DeGruy, *Post Traumatic Slave Syndrome: America's Legacy of Enduring Injury and Healing* (Milwaukie, OR: Uptone Press, 2005).
229 Carter, Robert T. "Racism and Psychological and Emotional Injury: Recognizing and Assessing Race-Based Traumatic Stress." *The Counseling Psychologist* 35, no. 1 (2007): 13-105.
230 Hortensia Amaro, Mariana Sanchez, Tara Bautista, and Robynn Cox, "Social Vulnerabilities for Substance Use: Stressors, Socially Toxic Environments, and Discrimination and Racism," *Neuropharmacology* 188 (2021): 108518, https://doi.org/10.1016/j.neuropharm.2021.108518. & Antonios Dakanalis et al., "The Association of Emotional Eating with Overweight/Obesity, Depression, Anxiety/Stress, and Dietary Patterns: A Review of the Current Clinical Evidence," *Nutrients* 15, no. 5 (2023): 1173, https://doi.org/10.3390/nu15051173. & Williams, David R., and Selina A. Mohammed. 2009. "Discrimination and Racial Disparities in Health: Evidence and Needed Research." *Journal of Behavioral Medicine* 32(1): 20-47. https://doi.org/10.1007/s10865-008-9185-0
231 Genesis Jacob, Scott C. Faber, Nicole Faber, Ashley Bartlett, Andrée J. Ouimet, and Monnica T. Williams, "A Systematic Review of Black People Coping With Racism: Approaches, Analysis, and Empowerment," *Perspectives on Psychological Science* 18, no. 2 (2023): 392-415, https://doi.org/10.1177/17456916221100509

Chapter 5
232 Brian G. Dias and Kerry J. Ressler, "Parental Olfactory Experience Influences Behavior and Neural Structure in Subsequent Generations," *Nature Neuroscience* 17, no. 1 (2014): 89-96, https://doi.org/10.1038/nn.3594
233 Ibid.
234 Rachel Yehuda and Alison Lehrner, "Intergenerational Transmission of Trauma Effects: Putative Role of Epigenetic Mechanisms," *World Psychiatry: Official Journal of the World Psychiatric Association (WPA)* 17, no. 3 (2018): 243-257, https://doi.org/10.1002/wps.20568
235 U.S. Department of Veterans Affairs, "Study Finds Epigenetic Changes in Children of Holocaust Survivors," *Office of Research & Development*, October 20, 2016, accessed February 4, 2021.

236 Ibid.
237 Ibid.
238 Rachel Yehuda and Alison Lehrner, "Intergenerational Transmission of Trauma Effects: Putative Role of Epigenetic Mechanisms," *World Psychiatry: Official Journal of the World Psychiatric Association (WPA)* 17, no. 3 (2018): 243-257, https://doi.org/10.1002/wps.20568
239 U.S. Department of Veterans Affairs, "Study Finds Epigenetic Changes in Children of Holocaust Survivors," *Office of Research & Development*, October 20, 2016, accessed February 4, 2021.
240 Bastiaan T. Heijmans et al., "Persistent Epigenetic Differences Associated with Prenatal Exposure to Famine in Humans," *Proceedings of the National Academy of Sciences of the United States of America* 105, no. 44 (2008): 17046-17049, https://doi.org/10.1073/pnas.0806560105.
241 Elmar W. Tobi et al., "DNA Methylation Differences after Exposure to Prenatal Famine Are Common and Timing- and Sex-Specific," *Human Molecular Genetics* 18, no. 21 (2009): 4046-4053, https://doi.org/10.1093/hmg/ddp353
242 Michael L. Blakey and Lesley M. Rankin-Hill, eds., *The Skeletal Biology of the New York African Burial Ground: Volume I, Part I* (Washington, DC: Howard University Press, 2009), 221-267.
243 Ibid, 121-125.
244 Ibid, 221-267.
245 National Institute of Environmental Health Sciences. "Retrieved April 1, 2021." *Developmental Origins of Health and Disease*. https://www.niehs.nih.gov/research/supported/health/developmental/index.cfm & Salvatore Lacagnina, "The Developmental Origins of Health and Disease (DOHaD)," *American Journal of Lifestyle Medicine* 14, no. 1 (2019): 47-50, https://doi.org/10.1177/1559827619879694 & Amanda C. Haugen et al., "Evolution of DOHaD: The Impact of Environmental Health Sciences," *Journal of Developmental Origins of Health and Disease* 6, no. 2 (2015): 55-64, https://doi.org/10.1017/S2040174414000580
246 Ibid.
247 James W. Collins Jr., Richard J. David, Arden Handler, Stephen Wall, and Steven Andes, "Very Low Birthweight in African American Infants: The Role of Maternal Exposure to Interpersonal Racial Discrimination," *American Journal of Public Health* 94, no. 12 (2004): 2132-2138, https://doi.org/10.2105/AJPH.94.12.2132.
248 Christopher W. Kuzawa and Elizabeth Sweet, "Epigenetics and the Embodiment of Race: Developmental Origins of US Racial Disparities in Cardiovascular Health," *American Journal of Human Biology* 21, no. 1 (2009): 2-15, https://doi.org/10.1002/ajhb.20822.

Chapter 6
249 Elizabeth Blackburn and Elissa Epel, The Telomere Effect: A Revolutionary Approach to Living Younger, Healthier, Longer (New York: Grand Central Publishing, 2017).

Endnotes

250 Gen Li et al., "Understanding the Protective Effect of Social Support on Depression Symptomatology from a Longitudinal Network Perspective," BMJ Mental Health 26, no. 1 (2023): e300802, https://doi.org/10.1136/bmjment-2023-300802
251 Ning Xia and Huige Li, "Loneliness, Social Isolation, and Cardiovascular Health," Antioxidants & Redox Signaling 28, no. 9 (2018): 837–851, https://doi.org/10.1089/ars.2017.7312 & Julianne Holt-Lunstad et al., "Loneliness and Social Isolation as Risk Factors for Mortality: A Meta-Analytic Review," Perspectives on Psychological Science 10, no. 2 (2015): 227–237, https://doi.org/10.1177/1745691614568352
252 Ingvild Oxås Henriksen et al., "The Role of Self-Esteem in the Development of Psychiatric Problems: A Three-Year Prospective Study in a Clinical Sample of Adolescents," Child and Adolescent Psychiatry and Mental Health 11 (2017): 68, https://doi.org/10.1186/s13034-017-0207-y
253 Gen Li et al., "Understanding the Protective Effect of Social Support on Depression Symptomatology from a Longitudinal Network Perspective," BMJ Mental Health 26, no. 1 (2023): e300802, https://doi.org/10.1136/bmjment-2023-300802
254 Grace Jacob et al., "A Systematic Review of Black People Coping With Racism: Approaches, Analysis, and Empowerment," Perspectives on Psychological Science 18, no. 2 (2023): 392–415, https://doi.org/10.1177/17456916221100509
255 Arline T. Geronimus, Weathering: The Extraordinary Stress of Ordinary Life in an Unjust Society (New York: Little, Brown Spark, 2023), 77-78.
256 On the Shoulder of Giants, "We Devalue Blackness For Individualism, Dr. Barbara Sizemore Lecture," April 1, 2025 https://www.youtube.com/watch?v=5Sf8FiaTOv8
257 Dhruv Khullar and Dave A. Chokshi, "Health, Income, and Poverty: Where We Are and What Could Help," Health Affairs Health Policy Brief, October 4, 2018,
258 Originally quoted as "broken men" adjusted to make language more gender inclusive.
259 Anthony L. Burrow et al., "The Role of Purpose in the Stress Process: A Homeostatic Account," Journal of Research in Personality 108 (February 2024): 104444, https://doi.org/10.1016/j.jrp.2023.104444
260 American Psychiatric Association, "Purpose in Life Can Lead to Less Stress, Better Mental Well-Being," APA Blogs, December 7, 2023, accessed April 28, 2025, https://www.psychiatry.org/news-room/apa-blogs/purpose-in-life-less-stress-better-mental-health
261 Patrick L. Hill and Nicholas A. Turiano, "Purpose in Life as a Predictor of Mortality Across Adulthood," Psychological Science 25, no. 7 (2014): 1482-1486, https://doi.org/10.1177/0956797614531799.
262 Girija Kaimal, Kendra Ray, and Juan Muniz, "Reduction of Cortisol Levels and Participants' Responses Following Art Making," Art Therapy: Journal of the American Art Therapy Association 33, no. 2 (2016): 74–80, https://doi.org/10.1080/07421656.2016.1166832 & Daisy Fancourt and Saoirse Finn, Health Evidence Network Synthesis Report, No. 67: What Is the Evidence on the Role of the Arts in Improving Health and Well-Being? A Scoping Review (Copenhagen: WHO Regional Office for Europe, 2019).

263 Dominique Lambright, "Why Black People Should Be Using Music to Boost Brain Health," BlackDoctor.org, March 7, 2025, accessed May 2, 2025, https://blackdoctor.org/why-black-people-should-be-using-music-to-boost-brain-health/

264 Giancarlo Lucchetti, Harold G. Koenig, and Alessandra L. G. Lucchetti, "Spirituality, Religiousness, and Mental Health: A Review of the Current Scientific Evidence," *World Journal of Clinical Cases* 9, no. 26 (2021): 7620–7631, https://doi.org/10.12998/wjcc.v9.i26.7620

265 Luis J. Dominguez, Nicola Veronese, and Mario Barbagallo, "The Link between Spirituality and Longevity," *Aging Clinical and Experimental Research* 36, no. 1 (2024): 32, https://doi.org/10.1007/s40520-023-02684-5.

Chapter 7

266 Julie Corliss, "Breathing Exercises to Lower Your Blood Pressure: A Regular Breathing Practice May Reduce Blood Pressure as Much as Taking Medication," *Harvard Health Publishing*, September 1, 2023, accessed May 2, 2025, https://www.health.harvard.edu/heart-health/breathing-exercises-to-lower-your-blood-pressure

267 S. Chaitanya et al., "Effect of Resonance Breathing on Heart Rate Variability and Cognitive Functions in Young Adults: A Randomised Controlled Study," *Cureus* 14, no. 2 (2022): e22187, https://doi.org/10.7759/cureus.22187

268 U.S. Department of Health & Human Services, *Office of Minority Health*, "Asthma and Black/African Americans," accessed January 30, 2025, https://minorityhealth.hhs.gov/asthma-and-blackafrican-americans

269 Eddie Weitzberg and Jon O. Lundberg, "Humming Greatly Increases Nasal Nitric Oxide," *American Journal of Respiratory and Critical Care Medicine* 166, no. 2 (2002): 144–145, https://doi.org/10.1164/rccm.200202-138BC

270 Nan Zhang et al., "Effects of Dehydration and Rehydration on Cognitive Performance and Mood among Male College Students in Cangzhou, China: A Self-Controlled Trial," *International Journal of Environmental Research and Public Health* 16, no. 11 (2019): 1891, https://doi.org/10.3390/ijerph16111891

271 U.S. Department of Health & Human Services, *Office of Minority Health*, " Heart Disease and Black/African Americans," accessed April 30, 2025, https://minorityhealth.hhs.gov/heart-disease-and-blackafrican-americans

272 UChicago Medicine, "Heart Disease and Racial Disparities: Why Heart Disease Is More Common in Black Patients and How to Prevent It," *UChicago Medicine*, February 26, 2021, https://www.uchicagomedicine.org/forefront/heart-and-vascular-articles/heart-disease-and-racial-disparities

273 Christopher Borden et al., "Black Patients Equally Benefit From Renal Genetics Evaluation but Substantial Barriers in Access Exist," *Kidney International Reports* 8, no. 10 (2023): 2068–2076, https://doi.org/10.1016/j.ekir.2023.07.007

274 U.S. Department of Health & Human Services, *Office of Minority Health*, " Diabetes and Black/African Americans," accessed May 6, 2025, https://minorityhealth.hhs.gov/diabetes-and-blackafrican-americans

Endnotes

275 National Institutes of Health, "Racial Disparities in Stroke Incidence and Death," *NIH Research Matters*, June 21, 2016, accessed January 30, 2025, https://www.nih.gov/news-events/nih-research-matters/racial-disparities-stroke-incidence-death

276 McKinsey & Company, "Too Many Black Americans Live in Food Deserts," *McKinsey & Company*, September 9, 2021, accessed March 31, 2025, https://www.mckinsey.com/featured-insights/sustainable-inclusive-growth/charts/too-many-black-americans-live-in-food-deserts

277 Keith Pinckard, Kyle K. Baskin, and Kristin I. Stanford, "Effects of Exercise to Improve Cardiovascular Health," *Frontiers in Cardiovascular Medicine* 6 (2019): 69, https://doi.org/10.3389/fcvm.2019.00069 & Md Nazmul Hossain et al., "The Impact of Exercise on Depression: How Moving Makes Your Brain and Body Feel Better," *Physical Activity and Nutrition* 28, no. 2 (2024): 43-51, https://doi.org/10.20463/pan.2024.0015

278 American Heart Association, "High Blood Pressure Among Black People," *American Heart Association*, accessed March 31, 2025, https://www.heart.org/en/health-topics/high-blood-pressure/know-your-risk-factors-for-high-blood-pressure/high-blood-pressure-among-black-people

279 John Elflein, "Adult Obesity Rates in the U.S. by Race/Ethnicity 2023," *Statista*, November 28, 2024, https://www.statista.com/statistics/207436/overweight-and-obesity-rates-for-adults-by-ethnicity/

280 NAMI California, "Mental Health in Black Communities: Challenges, Resources, Community Voices," accessed May 6, 2025, https://namica.org/mental-health-challenges-in-african-american-communities/

281 Xiaoning Huang et al., "Age at Diagnosis of Hypertension by Race and Ethnicity in the US From 2011 to 2020," *JAMA Cardiology* 7, no. 9 (2022): 986-987, https://doi.org/10.1001/jamacardio.2022.2345 & U.S. Department of Health & Human Services, Office of Minority Health, " Stroke and Black/African Americans," accessed May 6, 2025, https://minorityhealth.hhs.gov/stroke-and-blackafrican-americans

282 Eddie L. Hackler III, Naomi M. Hamburg, and Khendi T. White Solaru, "Racial and Ethnic Disparities in Peripheral Artery Disease," Circulation Research 128, no. 12 (2021): e246–e257, https://doi.org/10.1161/CIRCRESAHA.121.318243

283 National Institutes of Health, "Racial Disparities in Stroke Incidence and Death," *NIH Research Matters*, June 21, 2016, Accessed May 6, 2025, https://www.nih.gov/news-events/nih-research-matters/racial-disparities-stroke-incidence-death

284 Thomas D. Sequist et al., "Differences in Specialist Consultations for Cardiovascular Disease by Race, Ethnicity, Gender, Insurance Status, and Site of Primary Care," *Circulation* 119, no. 18 (2009): 2463-2470, https://doi.org/10.1161/CIRCULATIONAHA.108.825133

285 Mohammad Jalalyazdi et al., "Effect of Hibiscus Sabdariffa on Blood Pressure in Patients with Stage 1 Hypertension," *Journal of Advanced Pharmaceutical Technology & Research* 10, no. 3 (2019): 107-111, https://doi.org/10.4103/japtr.JAPTR_402_18

286 Patricia M. White et al., "Advancing Health Equity: The Association of Black Gastroenterologists and Hepatologists," *Nature Reviews Gastroenterology & Hepatology* 18, no. 7 (2021): 449-450, https://doi.org/10.1038/s41575-021-00464-y.

287 Ibid.

288 U.S. Department of Health & Human Services, *Office of Minority Health*, " Diabetes and Black/African Americans," accessed May 6, 2025, https://minorityhealth.hhs.gov/diabetes-and-blackafrican-americans

289 Harriet A. Washington, *A Terrible Thing to Waste: Environmental Racism and Its Assault on the American Mind* (New York: Little, Brown Spark, 2019).

290 National Kidney Foundation, *Health Disparities*, accessed May 7, 2025, https://www.kidney.org/get-involved/advocate/legislative-priorities/health-disparities

291 Perri Zeitz Ruckart et al., "The Flint Water Crisis: A Coordinated Public Health Emergency Response and Recovery Initiative," *Journal of Public Health Management and Practice* 25, suppl. 1 (2019): S84-S90, https://doi.org/10.1097/PHH.0000000000000871

292 Tawainna Houston, *Detox-Style: Creating a Healthy Lifestyle Through Daily Holistic Detoxification Practices* (North Charleston, SC: CreateSpace Independent Publishing Platform, 2016).

293 Michael A. Grandner et al., "Sleep Disparity, Race/Ethnicity, and Socioeconomic Position," *Sleep Medicine* 18 (2016): 7-18, https://doi.org/10.1016/j.sleep.2015.01.020

294 Abhishek Pandey et al., "Linking Sleep to Hypertension: Greater Risk for Blacks," *International Journal of Hypertension* 2013 (2013): Article ID 436502, https://doi.org/10.1155/2013/436502

295 Michael A. Grandner et al., "Sleep Disparity, Race/Ethnicity, and Socioeconomic Position," *Sleep Medicine* 18 (2016): 7-18, https://doi.org/10.1016/j.sleep.2015.01.020

296 Maurice J. Chery and Rhoda Moise, "Public Health Implications of Sleep Health in Black Americans Using the Socio-Ecological Model and a Life-Course Approach: A Systematic Literature Review," *Social Sciences & Humanities Open* 10, no. 4 (2024): 101017, https://doi.org/10.1016/j.ssaho.2024.101017

297 Martha E. Billings et al., "Disparities in Sleep Health and Potential Intervention Models: A Focused Review," *Chest* 159, no. 3 (2021): 1232-1240, https://doi.org/10.1016/j.chest.2020.09.249

298 George M. Slavich and Michael R. Irwin, "From Stress to Inflammation and Major Depressive Disorder: A Social Signal Transduction Theory of Depression," *Psychological Bulletin* 140, no. 3 (2014): 780, https://doi.org/10.1037/a0035302 & Neha Singh et al., "Inflammation and Cancer," *Annals of African Medicine* 18, no. 3 (2019): 121-126, https://doi.org/10.4103/aam.aam_56_18

299 Farida B. Ahmad, Jodi A. Cisewski, and Robert N. Anderson, "Mortality in the United States – Provisional Data, 2023," *Morbidity and Mortality Weekly Report* 73, no. 31 (August 8, 2024): 682-686, U.S. Centers for Disease Control and Prevention, https://

Endnotes

www.cdc.gov/mmwr/mmwr_continuingEducation.html
300 Cecilia de Luca and Jerrold M. Olefsky, "Inflammation and Insulin Resistance," *FEBS Letters* 582, no. 1 (2008): 97–105, https://doi.org/10.1016/j.febslet.2007.11.057
301 Connor D. Martz et al., "Incident Racial Discrimination Predicts Elevated C-Reactive Protein in the Black Women's Experiences Living with Lupus (BeWELL) Study," *Brain, Behavior, and Immunity* 112 (2023): 77–84, https://doi.org/10.1016/j.bbi.2023.06.004
302 Huazhen Zhao et al., "Inflammation and Tumor Progression: Signaling Pathways and Targeted Intervention," *Signal Transduction and Targeted Therapy* 6, no. 263 (2021), https://doi.org/10.1038/s41392-021-00658-5
303 Margarita Vasquez Reyes, "The Disproportional Impact of COVID-19 on African Americans," *Health and Human Rights* 22, no. 2 (2020): 299–307.
304 Syreen Goulmamine, "Elevating the Impacts of Autoimmune Disease and Black Women's Health," *Society for Women's Health Research*, February 26, 2024, accessed May 7, 2025, https://swhr.org/elevating-the-impacts-of-autoimmune-disease-and-black-womens-health/
305 Ronald L. Simons et al., "Discrimination, Segregation, and Chronic Inflammation: Testing the Weathering Explanation for the Poor Health of Black Americans," *Developmental Psychology* 54, no. 10 (2018): 1993–2006, https://doi.org/10.1037/dev0000511
306 Jiaquan Xu, Sherry L. Murphy, Kenneth D. Kochanek, and Elizabeth Arias, Deaths: Final Data for 2019, *National Vital Statistics Reports*, vol. 70, no. 8 (Hyattsville, MD: National Center for Health Statistics, July 26, 2021). https://www.cdc.gov/nchs/data/nvsr/nvsr70/nvsr70-08-508.pdf
307 Wizdom Powell et al., "Medical Mistrust, Racism, and Delays in Preventive Health Screening Among African-American Men," *Behavioral Medicine* 45, no. 2 (2019): 102–117, https://doi.org/10.1080/08964289.2019.1585327
308 Bruce N. Ames, William B. Grant, and Walter C. Willett, "Does the High Prevalence of Vitamin D Deficiency in African Americans Contribute to Health Disparities?" *Nutrients* 13, no. 2 (2021): 499, https://doi.org/10.3390/nu13020499
309 Maryam Hajhashemi et al., "The Effect of Vitamin D Supplementation on the Size of Uterine Leiomyoma in Women with Vitamin D Deficiency," *Caspian Journal of Internal Medicine* 10, no. 2 (2019): 125–131, https://doi.org/10.22088/cjim.10.2.125.
310 David R. Williams, "Stress and the Mental Health of Populations of Color: Advancing Our Understanding of Race-Related Stressors," *Journal of Health and Social Behavior* 59, no. 4 (2018): 466–485, https://doi.org/10.1177/0022146518814251
311 Mathias Berger and Zoltán Sarnyai, "'More than Skin Deep': Stress Neurobiology and Mental Health Consequences of Racial Discrimination," *Stress* 18, no. 1 (2014): 1–10, https://doi.org/10.3109/10253890.2014.989204
312 Tanya M. Spruill et al., "Association Between High Perceived Stress Over Time and

Incident Hypertension in Black Adults: Findings From the Jackson Heart Study," *Journal of the American Heart Association* 8, no. 21 (2019): e012139, originally published October 16, 2019, https://doi.org/10.1161/JAHA.119.012139

313 George M. Slavich and Michael R. Irwin, "From Stress to Inflammation and Major Depressive Disorder: A Social Signal Transduction Theory of Depression," *Psychological Bulletin* 140, no. 3 (2014): 780, https://doi.org/10.1037/a0035302

314 Concetta Gardi et al., "A Short Mindfulness Retreat Can Improve Biological Markers of Stress and Inflammation," *Psychoneuroendocrinology* 135 (January 2022): 105579, https://doi.org/10.1016/j.psyneuen.2021.105579

315 Waranya Turakitwanakan, Chatchada Mekseepralard, and Pimonpan Busarakumtragul, "Effects of Mindfulness Meditation on Serum Cortisol of Medical Students," *Journal of the Medical Association of Thailand* = Chotmaihet Thangphaet 96, suppl. 1 (2013): S90–S95 & Rui Wu et al., "Brief Mindfulness Meditation Improves Emotion Processing," *Frontiers in Neuroscience* 13 (2019): 1074, https://doi.org/10.3389/fnins.2019.01074

316 U.S. Department of Health and Human Services, *Our Epidemic of Loneliness and Isolation: The U.S. Surgeon General's Advisory on the Healing Effects of Social Connection and Community* (Washington, DC: U.S. Department of Health and Human Services, 2023), https://www.hhs.gov/sites/default/files/surgeon-general-social-connection-advisory.pdf

317 Zulqarnain Javed et al., "Race, Racism, and Cardiovascular Health: Applying a Social Determinants of Health Framework to Racial/Ethnic Disparities in Cardiovascular Disease," *Circulation: Cardiovascular Quality and Outcomes* 15, no. 1 (2022): e007917, https://doi.org/10.1161/CIRCOUTCOMES.121.007917

318 "Prevention Is the Cure," as told to Victoria Uwumarogie, *Essence*, January/February 2025.

319 American Diabetes Association, "Statistics About Diabetes," *American Diabetes Association*, accessed May 8, 2025, https://diabetes.org/about-diabetes/statistics/about-diabetes

320 Sharla M. Fett *Working Cures: Healing, Health, and Power on Southern Slave Plantations*. Chapel Hill: University of North Carolina Press, 2002.

INDEX

A
Acupuncturists 291
aerobic exercise 240, 245
affirmations 198
Affordable Care Act (ACA) 101
affordable housing 87, 88, 121
African-American Credit Union Coalition 207
African dance 93, 214, 242
African Proverb 186
Afrofuturism 213, 214
aggressive Black man 158
agricultural runoff 119
air pollution 85, 119, 120, 122, 153, 226, 246, 271
Alternative Providers 288
American Dream 115
amputations 149
ancestor veneration 58
angry Black woman 158
antebellum South 27, 28, 76
apoptosis 151
arthritis 45, 47, 49, 168, 240, 241, 263, 269
Assin Manso Slave River 40
asthma 87, 120, 121, 169, 170, 172, 226, 256, 319
Atlantic Ocean 41, 44
Autoimmune 264, 269, 322
autonomy 18, 39, 56, 59, 61, 62, 65, 67, 74, 80, 108, 157, 196, 197, 199, 208, 239

B
Bacon, Nathaniel 21
Bacon's Rebellion 21, 23, 24, 36
Bethune, Mary McLeod 208
biological aging 116, 145, 152
biology of stress 140
Biosphere 2 295

Black bodies 10, 11, 18, 22, 26, 33, 35, 46, 50, 95, 99, 100, 125, 141, 174, 283, 289, 294
Black Business Directories 206
Black churches 185, 193, 202
Black Codes 78, 114, 124, 180, 196
Black college graduates 110
Black Diseases 28
BlackDoctor.org 292, 318
Black Emotional and Mental Health Collective (BEAM) 292
Black Lives Matter 13, 180, 192, 200, 218
Black Panther Party 208, 280
Black Star Network 196
Black Urban Growers 202, 237
branding 66
breast cancer 102, 145, 151
Breathwork 227
breeding 38, 41, 46, 60, 67, 71
British Whitehall studies 107, 109
Brown, James 186
Brown v. Board of Education 89
brutal beatings 65
Buy Black movement 197

C
Cachexia Africana 28
calcium 29, 53
Caldwell, Charles 27, 35, 300
call-and-response 48, 217
Cancer Alley 120, 311
Cancer Screenings 288
Cape Coast Castle 40
cardiac catheterization 103
cardiovascular aging 146
cardiovascular disease 86, 96, 127, 130, 136, 140, 143, 147, 149, 155, 166, 169, 193, 229, 234, 240, 244, 248, 268, 273, 287, 288

CAREN's Act 126
Cartwright, Samuel A 28, 301
castration 67
chants 48
Chattel slavery 50
Child mortality 168
Chiropractors 291
Chitlin' Circuit 186
Cholesterol 287
Christianity 58, 59, 62, 217
Chronic pain 47
chronic stress 25, 85, 87, 94, 98, 106, 107, 108, 111, 116, 120, 125, 127, 133, 144, 145, 148, 149, 150, 152, 154, 155, 156, 157, 161, 163, 164, 168, 172, 174, 188, 205, 221, 226, 259, 268, 273, 274, 279, 290
Chronic stress 46, 93, 108, 136, 143, 144, 145, 148, 149, 150, 152, 153, 156, 164, 246, 248, 253, 261, 265, 269, 271, 274
Circulation 103, 244, 245, 246, 247, 248, 309, 320, 323
Civil Rights 79, 181, 186, 192, 200, 208
Coates, Ta-Nehisi 215
coded language 48, 129
code-switching 279
cognitive decline 156, 214, 244, 245, 251, 287
cognitive impairments 157
collective work songs 48
collectivism 186
colonial 18, 21, 22, 24, 25, 35, 48, 167
Colonoscopy
    Colonoscopies 253
colorectal 249, 250, 264
Colorism 71
Complementary Providers 288
Cone, James 218
    God of the Oppressed 218
congestive heart failure 103
connection 57, 58, 59, 62, 63, 64, 65, 133, 161, 179, 188, 189, 214, 220, 243, 249, 278, 280, 296, 323
Coogler, Ryan 215
cotton 45, 51

COVID-19 13, 104, 150, 268, 269, 270, 285, 322
critical developmental windows 170
Crown Act 106
CRP 144, 152, 287
cruciferous vegetables 255, 264
cultural beliefs 58
cultural erasure 57, 65, 91
cultural knowledge 64, 79, 281
cultural preservation 51, 55, 59, 179, 180, 208, 213, 289
cycle of poverty 92, 116
cytokines 264, 266, 269, 274

D

Dance 58
dark leafy greens 237, 245, 247, 255
degenerative joint diseases 45
Degruy, Joy
    Post-Traumatic Slave Syndrome (PTSS) 159
DeGruy, Joy 159, 312, 316
delayed diagnoses 99, 102, 152, 292
Dental Check-Ups 288
dental enamel hypoplasia 168
depression 71, 85, 94, 98, 111, 116, 134, 135, 156, 159, 160, 163, 164, 165, 170, 192, 197, 201, 205, 209, 213, 218, 230, 234, 240, 251, 260, 273, 274, 278, 279
Detoxification 254, 255, 256, 257, 258, 321, 333, 334
Developmental Origins of Health and Disease (DOHaD) 169, 317
diabetes 10, 36, 85, 93, 96, 98, 102, 108, 127, 140, 143, 144, 145, 148, 155, 169, 171, 174, 201, 205, 230, 234, 235, 239, 240, 242, 244, 245, 249, 250, 251, 260, 263, 268, 270, 274, 287, 288, 290, 294, 308, 314, 319, 321, 323
    insulin resistance 107, 148, 155, 170, 252, 260
Diabetes Screening 287
Digestion 249, 250, 251, 252
disease vulnerabilities 36, 108

INDEX

disinvestment 84, 86, 89, 96, 122, 127, 129, 206, 212, 294
displaced 86, 118
DNA 44, 140, 162, 164, 166, 264, 317
FKBP5 164
IGF2 166
doctor-patient relationship 102
Doll Test 133
    Kenneth and Mamie Clark 133
dominant culture 25
Drapetomania 28
drumming 58, 214
Du Bois, W.E.B. 208
Dutch Hunger Winter 140, 166, 167, 168
DuVernay, Ava 213
dysentery 42

E

Early detection 102, 283, 286, 287
economic 18, 20, 22, 23, 26, 45, 47, 56, 61, 67, 69, 71, 75, 76, 78, 83, 84, 85, 86, 88, 89, 92, 96, 97, 99, 100, 106, 111, 112, 113, 114, 115, 116, 122, 124, 129, 131, 140, 143, 144, 147, 149, 150, 152, 153, 172, 180, 185, 186, 189, 192, 197, 200, 202, 203, 204, 205, 206, 207, 208, 212, 214, 217, 221, 254, 259, 265, 273, 277, 279, 282, 283, 315
Elder Playdates 195
emancipation 11, 29, 68, 75, 78, 80, 100, 124, 180, 185, 200, 239, 259
emasculation 65, 68
emotional dysregulation 158, 159
endorphins 276
environmental 36, 49, 85, 117, 118, 119, 120, 121, 122, 123, 128, 137, 146, 149, 152, 153, 162, 166, 169, 170, 171, 172, 173, 174, 175, 193, 203, 226, 228, 231, 239, 244, 248, 249, 254, 255, 256, 258, 259, 261, 262, 263, 268, 269, 272, 285, 294
epigenetics
    acetophenone scent 163
    fear response 162, 163
Epigenetics 162, 163, 164, 317

Essence Magazine 285
essential service 150
Eurocentric beauty standards 106
executions 44, 60, 164
Eye Exams 288

F

family separations 63, 64, 165
Federal Housing Administration (FHA) 84
Fermented foods 250, 252, 271
Ferritin 287
fiber-rich diet 249
fibrinogen 144
fight-or-flight 146, 226, 273
Flint water crisis 118
Floyd, George 13, 125
Food as Medicine 234
food deserts 95, 96, 98, 137, 171, 251
food insecurity 97, 98, 149, 152, 171, 202, 249, 254, 268, 269
food swamps 95, 96, 98, 236
forced reproduction 11, 70
Franklin, Aretha 186
freedom 25, 28, 29, 36, 42, 56, 61, 68, 72, 77, 78, 79, 113, 116, 180, 184, 185, 189, 203, 217, 218, 231, 246, 290
Freedom Georgia Initiative 205
Freedom Schools 209

G

Garvey, Marcus 196, 208
Gastroesophageal Reflux Disease (GERD) 250
gene expression 162, 164, 167, 170, 174
generational trauma 33, 140, 160, 211
genetic line 175
gentrification 86, 87, 88, 192, 306
Geronimus, Arline 128, 145, 147
Ghana 39
GI Bill 114
Global warming 122
glucose 108, 142, 148, 149, 235, 250, 258, 287
Gone with the Wind 132
green spaces 122, 127, 239
grief 13, 39, 41, 43, 70, 154, 157, 160, 227, 280
grounding 178, 195, 209, 248, 273

Gut Dysbiosis 250

H

Harlem Renaissance 212
Harvard Implicit Association Test 132
HBCU 39
health disparities 32, 34, 39, 47, 52, 83, 85, 87, 88, 93, 95, 96, 97, 99, 111, 116, 118, 122, 127, 130, 136, 143, 147, 150, 152, 163, 167, 169, 172, 174, 192, 197, 200, 234, 236, 244, 249, 263, 267, 268, 269, 272, 295
health screenings 99, 108, 251, 253, 286, 292
Henrieta Lacks
    HeLa cell line 100
Henrietta Lacks 100
Herbalists 291
Herbs 248, 266
high-effort coping 147
High-Sensitivity C-Reactive Protein 287
hip-hop 182, 212
Hip-hop therapy 213
    rap 213
hippocampus 156
historical dehumanization 11, 39, 294
historical pain 71
historical trauma 36, 140, 156, 157, 159, 166, 168, 169, 173, 174, 187, 275, 278
Holocaust 140, 163, 164, 165, 168, 316, 317
home appraisals 115
    undervaluing homes 115
homeostasis 144, 182
Home Owners' Loan Corporation 84
Homocysteine 287
hormonal imbalances 148, 153, 254, 259, 273
Howard University 284, 303, 317, 332
Hughes, Langston 212
Hutu 24
Hydration 229, 230, 231, 232, 248, 255, 257, 266
hyper-sexualization 71
hypertension 10, 25, 36, 85, 86, 93, 96, 98, 108, 130, 136, 140, 143, 145, 146, 154, 155, 170, 171, 174, 193, 201, 205, 226, 227, 229, 230, 234, 235, 239, 240, 244, 245, 246, 248, 260, 263, 270, 273, 274, 287, 290, 291, 294
hypervigilance 157, 159, 261
hypothalamic-pituitary-adrenal (HPA) axis 142, 146, 151, 153, 164
hyptertension
    blood pressure 108, 142, 143, 146, 147, 154, 157, 170, 214, 225, 226, 230, 235, 239, 240, 244, 245, 246, 247, 260, 264, 274, 287

I

immune function 80, 143, 144, 149, 151, 164, 225, 239, 249, 259, 268, 269, 271, 273, 287
immunotherapy 152, 314
implicit bias 104, 112, 152
imprisonment 77, 114
inadequate treatment 99
indentured servants 22, 113
indoctrination 26
industrial zoning 120, 226
inferiority 10, 18, 19, 20, 21, 26, 27, 28, 29, 30, 31, 32, 37, 44, 57, 59, 68, 73, 76, 78, 80, 90, 131, 133, 134, 136, 159, 163, 188, 270, 294
infertility 153, 154, 314
inflammation 80, 136, 143, 144, 145, 148, 149, 150, 151, 152, 153, 156, 163, 165, 230, 235, 240, 241, 244, 246, 248, 249, 250, 251, 252, 254, 258, 259, 263, 264, 265, 266, 268, 269, 273, 274, 287, 291
internalized racism 134, 135, 136, 137
In Vitro Fertilization (IVF) 153
iron 29, 53, 168, 287

J

James, Sherman 146
Jim Crow 12, 78, 114, 124, 180, 187, 196
John Henryism 146, 147, 313
joint pain 263
joint stress 45

K

Karenga, Maulana Ron 187

INDEX

Kemetic 225
kidney disease 149, 229, 230, 255
kinship 55, 192, 200, 280

L

language 31, 57, 58, 59, 77, 213, 318
Lawrence, Jacob 212
lead contamination 85
learned helplessness 156, 159
learning disabilities 155
Lee, Spike 215
Lewis, Ananda 284
liberation 14, 62, 76, 79, 142, 196, 203, 208, 215, 216, 217, 218, 222, 231, 240
life expectancy 39, 72, 83, 99
low birth weight 154, 155
low birth weights 54, 98
low self-esteem 71
lupus 269
lymphatic 244, 245, 246, 254, 255, 258

M

macronutrients 52
magnesium 53, 262
maladaptive behaviors 161
maladaptive coping mechanisms 94, 116, 136
malaria 32
Malcolm X 208
malnutrition 29, 44, 52, 54, 70, 166, 167, 168, 234, 249
Malnutrition 46, 168
Mammy figures 132
Marginalization 97
Martin, Roland 196
mass incarceration 36, 172, 192
maternal mortality 35, 36, 70, 154, 201, 294
maternal mortality rate 35
Maternal stress 170
McMillan, Terry 213
Medical Advocacy 262
medical experimentation 11, 47, 100, 164
medical racism 27, 28, 31, 32, 33, 154, 197
Medical Racism 251, 265
mental distress 125, 249
mental health disorders 125, 273, 275

mental illness 28, 36
metabolic disease 47, 232
metabolic syndrome 148, 149, 260
Methylation 164, 317
microaggressions 93, 109, 143, 156, 160, 227, 274
microbiome 235, 236, 249, 250, 252, 265, 266
Middle Passage 41, 44, 302
Mindfulness 265, 274, 276, 323
minerals 52, 269
miscarriage 70, 154
mistrust 34, 63, 99, 100, 124, 152, 159, 270, 274, 284
mitigation 183
Mitigation
　mitigation 184
monogenism 30
Moore, Susan 104
Morton, Samuel 30
Morton, Samuel George 31, 301
Movement 79, 192, 196, 200, 208, 212, 214, 239, 240, 241, 242, 243, 258, 307
multiple sclerosis 269
muscle attachment sites 167
musculoskeletal disorders 47, 49
mutilation 60
Mutual aid societies 185

N

naming practices 59, 76
narrative 10, 18, 20, 24, 25, 26, 27, 33, 37, 44, 63, 68, 73, 74, 76, 77, 78, 80, 98, 111, 131, 132, 134, 161, 163, 167, 180, 184, 196, 199, 212, 223, 296
National Association for the Advancement of Colored People (NAACP) 217
National Institute of Environmental Health Sciences 169
native tongues 57
Naturopathic Doctors 290
Negro Motorist Green Book 185
neurodevelopmental disorders 155
neuroinflammation 156
neuropathy 149, 245

neurotoxicity 156
New York African Burial Ground 140, 167, 168, 303, 317
Niacin (B3) deficiency 53
nitric oxide 228, 247
Nott, Josiah 31, 32, 34
Nutrient-Dense Foods 251, 271
nutrition 38, 51, 52, 54, 55, 95, 97, 98, 99, 170, 171, 178, 209, 234, 235, 236, 238, 244, 253, 263, 283, 290
nutritional deficiencies 47, 169

O

obesity 91, 96, 102, 107, 127, 144, 145, 146, 147, 148, 154, 166, 170, 171, 229, 230, 232, 234, 235, 239, 240, 242, 249, 251, 260, 264, 313, 314, 320
Omega-3 fatty acids 245
oppression 18, 22, 23, 25, 29, 37, 39, 51, 56, 58, 61, 72, 73, 75, 76, 77, 78, 81, 111, 114, 120, 124, 131, 135, 136, 140, 144, 153, 157, 158, 159, 160, 163, 164, 167, 168, 173, 174, 178, 179, 182, 185, 188, 192, 195, 197, 200, 203, 208, 209, 212, 213, 214, 217, 218, 220, 221, 222, 223, 226, 234, 236, 238, 247, 254, 259, 268, 273, 277, 278, 282, 289
oral history 51, 59

P

pain management 28, 34, 103, 292
pancreatic cancer 249
particulate matter 120
Pay rate disparities 110
pellagra 53
Perry, Tyler 213
petrochemical plants 120
phenotypic plasticity 174
phrenology 27, 80
physical exploitation 18, 45, 167
physical tax 147
physical violation 60
pica 29
pit schools 79

plant-based 197, 218, 234, 245, 249, 251, 254, 288, 291
pneumonia 49, 269
Police Brutality 125
polycystic ovary syndrome (PCOS) 153
polygenism 30, 31, 32
porotic hyperostosis 54, 168
Post-Traumatic Stress Disorder (PTSD) 158
potassium 232, 235, 245, 247
Predatory lending 115
Preeclampsia 154, 315
pregnancy 46, 54, 98, 102, 153, 154, 155, 166, 167, 170
pregnancy and childbirth 46
premature aging 86, 145, 155, 263, 273
premature death 51, 120, 144, 167, 184, 290, 294
preterm births 98, 154, 155, 173
preventable 36, 99, 102, 293
Principles of Kwanzaa 187, 191
    Imani 217, 218, 219, 220
    Kujichagulia 196, 197, 198, 199
    Kuumba 212, 213, 214, 216
    Nguzo Saba 187, 191, 221, 222, 224
    Nia 208, 209, 210, 211
    Ujamaa 204, 206, 207, 221
    Ujima 200, 201, 202, 203, 221
    Umoja 192, 193, 195
prison-industrial complex 114
progesterone 153
pseudo 26, 30, 34, 36
    pseudoscience 27, 28, 31, 34, 80
pseudoscientific 11, 18, 28, 32, 33, 73
psychological distress 134, 135, 157, 158
psychological trauma 29, 47, 56, 60, 66, 67, 68, 70, 79, 247
psychological wounds 63, 64, 68
    psychosocial stress 146
psychosocial stressors 169
Public safety 123

R

racial hierarchy 18, 22, 23, 27, 30, 73, 74
racially restrictive covenants 84, 115

INDEX

racial policing 23
racial profiling 75, 124, 125, 157, 273
racial toxicity
    racially toxic 161
Rae, Issa 213
Rebounding 246, 255
Reconstruction era 204
Reconstruction-era 180
redlining 36, 84, 85, 88, 89, 95, 115, 172, 212
redwood trees 296
Regenerates 259
Religious practices 58
Reparations Task Force Report 113
representation 91, 104, 109, 136, 180, 181, 207, 215
reproduction 60, 65, 69, 70
reproductive health 32, 153, 154, 259
residential segregation 84
respiratory illnesses 85, 87, 122, 226
Rest 259, 260, 261, 262, 271
Rosenwald Schools 186
Rosewood 193, 204
Rwandan genocide 24

S

scientific racism 30, 31
sedentary 91, 239
Self-advocacy 197, 292
Self-Advocacy Strategies 292
self-care 35, 179, 198, 209, 210, 239, 241, 243, 277, 283, 288
self-governance 78
self-hatred 71
serotonin 240, 249, 251
Serum Iron Levels 287
service jobs 107
sexual exploitation 46, 65, 67, 69
sharecropping 113
Simone, Nina 212
Sims, James Marion 32, 34
Sizemore, Barbara 204, 318
Skeletal deformations 168
slave patrols 22
Sleep Hygiene 262

smallpox 42
social exclusion 25, 129, 147
social hierarchy 16, 22, 23, 25, 73
Social identity 131
Social Security Act of 1935 114
socioeconomic institution 39
Soul Fire Farm 201, 237
spirituals 48, 180, 212
stereotypes 28, 64, 73, 75, 78, 94, 132, 134, 135, 136, 196, 198
stigma 134, 274, 276
stigmatization 74
stillbirth 154
storytelling 58, 59, 76, 79, 180, 195, 209, 212, 213, 214, 216, 279
stress hormone 80, 150, 151, 163, 260, 273
stress hormones
    adrenaline 142, 146, 150
    cortisol 85, 142, 144, 145, 146, 148, 149, 150, 151, 153, 156, 163, 164, 213, 214, 226, 246, 253, 260, 264, 269, 274, 276, 278, 279
stress management 262, 272, 273, 283
stress reduction 178, 218, 226, 248, 264, 271, 274, 279
stress response 11, 136, 142, 143, 144, 145, 146, 149, 173, 236, 259
Strokes 146
structural barriers 11, 98, 133, 136, 147, 149, 159, 178, 183, 208
Structural barriers 110
Structural racism 12
sugar 45, 149, 160, 168, 235, 236, 237, 240, 247, 249, 250, 251, 262, 264, 265
suicide 43, 44, 63
surnames 57
surveillance 22, 46, 60, 74, 126
sympathetic nervous system 146, 274
systemic discrimination 124, 132

T

telomeres 145, 151, 187
The Birth of a Nation 132
Thyroid Levels 288

tobacco 45, 160
tooth decay 168
toxic stress 47
toxic waste 118, 122
Trans-Atlantic Slave Trade 44
transgenerational health 85, 168, 173
transportation inequities 129, 130
trauma 11, 12, 37, 39, 44, 51, 63, 64, 68, 80, 140, 141, 156, 157, 158, 162, 163, 164, 165, 167, 169, 172, 174, 185, 188, 192, 194, 200, 201, 208, 209, 213, 216, 221, 227, 236, 241, 244, 247, 273, 277, 278, 281, 294, 295, 297
tuberculosis 49
Tulsa's Black Wall Street 204
Tuskegee Institute 217
Tuskegee Study of Untreated Syphilis in the Negro Male 100
Tutsis 24
typhoid fever 42

U

Ubuntu 188, 296
unarmed Black 125
underfunded healthcare 99
Underground Railroad 192, 196
under-resourced 36
unemployment rates 105
unfertilized eggs 174
Urban heat islands 122

V

violence 18, 24, 34, 39, 40, 43, 45, 46, 61, 65, 66, 67, 68, 69, 71, 73, 74, 77, 79, 80, 123, 124, 125, 132, 140, 153, 157, 163, 168, 178, 193, 200, 205, 212, 275
visualization 276
vitamin D 53, 270, 285, 287
Vitamin D Levels 287
vitamins 52, 53, 269

W

Walker, Kara 215
Washington, Booker T. 217
water contamination 119, 229
weakened immune systems 51, 54
weathering 128, 145, 274
Weathering
    Weathering Hypothesis 155
West Africa 39, 53, 289
whip 44, 60, 68, 77
whiteness 22, 23, 25, 73, 75, 133
white superiority 30, 80
white supremacy 21, 69, 73, 76
World Health Organization 38, 83, 302

Y

Yehuda, Rachel 164, 316, 317
yellow fever 32
yoga 241, 258, 266, 276

ABOUT THE AUTHOR

Dr. Tawainna Houston is a licensed naturopathic physician and leading expert in systemic health equity and chronic disease prevention, with over two decades of experience addressing the historical, biological, and transgenerational roots of illness in Black communities. As the founder of Black CELL Consulting, she delivers culturally centered wellness education to Black professionals, guiding them through the layered impact of racial toxicity, environmental stressors, and structural inequities on their health and well-being.

Blending expertise in sociology, counseling, and natural medicine, Dr. Houston equips individuals and communities with practical tools for stress mitigation and life-affirming wellness practices, helping them shift from survival to sustainable thriving. She holds a Doctorate in Naturopathic Medicine from National University of Health Sciences, a Master of Divinity in Pastoral Care & Counseling from Princeton Seminary, and a Bachelor's degree in Sociology from Howard University, grounding her work in both scientific rigor and cultural insight.

Dr. Houston is the best-selling Amazon author of *Black Wellness Barriers: Understanding the Root Cause of Disease Vulnerabilities as a Pathway Towards Restoring Health*, an Amazon #1 New Release in Hypertension. Other published work includes *Detox-Style: Creating a Healthy Lifestyle Through Daily Holistic Detoxification Practices*. Her voice and expertise have been featured in newspapers, urban radio stations, and in multiple podcast interviews exploring topics in health equity and cultural wellness.

She served multiple years as an adjunct instructor teaching cultural competency in clinical care to medical students, preparing the next generation of healthcare professionals to practice with greater empathy and equity. In addition to her work with Black CELL Consulting, Dr. Houston is the founder of Journey of Wellness Natural Medicine Center, a virtual holistic health consulting practice.

A recognized thought leader in cultural wellness and Black health advocacy, she has presented at medical conferences, served on international medical service trips, and held leadership roles, including Co-Chair of the Diversity, Equity & Inclusion Committee for the American Association of Naturopathic Physicians (AANP). With deep poise and dedication, Dr. Houston continues to inspire through her writing, speaking, and unwavering commitment to empowering others with culturally grounded, holistic care.

Website: https://blackcellconsulting.com

LinkedIN: https://www.linkedin.com/in/drthoustonnd/

ABOUT THE AUTHOR

For guided discussion questions and reflection activities tailored for Black readers, People of Color, White allies, healthcare, and mental health professionals, visit:
https://wellnessedu.blackcellconsulting.com
to access your FREE REFLECTION GUIDE.

ALSO BY DR. TAWAINNA HOUSTON

DETOX-STYLE

Creating A Healthy Lifestyle Through Daily Holistic Detoxification Practices

"Powerful" and "transformative," Detox-Style equips you with the critical awareness needed to understand how daily toxin exposure contributes to disease. By presenting detoxification as a lifestyle—"a Detox-style"—this book reveals how the body naturally eliminates toxins and offers actionable strategies to support this process. Without proper detox, the risk of disease escalates. Detox-Style empowers readers to reduce harmful exposures and adopt holistic detoxification practices for lasting health.

Available on: amazon.com

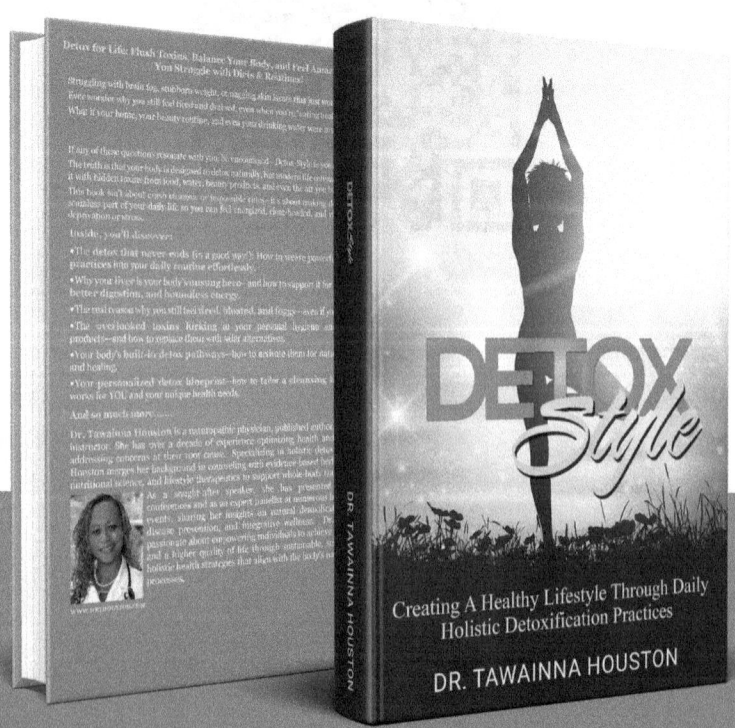

www.ingramcontent.com/pod-product-compliance
Lightning Source LLC
Chambersburg PA
CBHW060451030426
42337CB00015B/1547